S0-CAT-625

The Brain Boost:

A Practical Guide to Brain Health

Kathy N. Johnson, PhD, CMC

James H. Johnson, PhD

Lily Sarafan, MS

The information contained in this book is intended to provide helpful information on the subject addressed. It is not intended to serve as a replacement for professional medical advice. Any use of the information in this book is at the reader's discretion. The authors and publisher specifically disclaim any and all liability arising directly or indirectly from the use or application of any material contained in this book. A health care professional should be consulted regarding your specific situation.

All Rights Reserved. No part of this book may be used or reproduced in any matter without the written permission of the Publisher. Printed in the United States of America. For information, address Home Care Press, 148 Hawthorne Avenue, Palo Alto, CA 94301.

ISBN 978-0-9857236-4-4

Copyright © 2014 Home Care Assistance, Inc.

OTHER BOOKS BY THE AUTHORS

Happy to 102: The Best Kept Secrets to a Long and Happy Life

The Handbook of Live-in Care: A Guide for Caregivers

From Hospital to Home Care: A Step by Step Guide to Providing Care to Patients Post Hospitalization

The Five Senses: A Sensible Guide to Sensory Loss

Mind Over Gray Matter: A New Approach to Dementia Care

The Senior Sleep Solution: A Guide to Improving Sleep in Later Life

ACKNOWLEDGMENTS

This book is dedicated to the researchers around the globe working to increase our understanding of cognitive health. We hope that presenting practical lifestyle tips for brain fitness will encourage men and women of every age to embrace a brain-healthy lifestyle.

This book is inspired by the thousands of clients with whom we work each day. They motivate us to be better family members, friends, clinicians, social workers, care managers, caregivers and neighbors.

TABLE OF CONTENTS

CHAPTER 1

INTRODUCTION: THE BRAIN AND DEMENTIA

We all know that the brain is an incredibly complex organ. But many of us may not appreciate the full extent of that complexity until we are faced with challenges in cognitive health, either in ourselves or in someone we love.

We are born with 100 billion brain cells that are capable of making trillions of connections with each other. Those connections create pathways that contribute to who we are and control what we do. As we progress from infancy through adolescence and into adulthood, a certain amount of "pruning" takes place and unused pathways are discarded, analogous to how the scaffolding around a new building gets dismantled. Once we hit our mid-twenties, the brain's aging process commences, and we start to lose neurons, resulting in subtle declines in certain cognitive abilities – we can become less mentally flexible and take more time to process information. In various neurodegenerative diseases, the loss of neurons and neural connections is greater and results in cognitive detriments severe enough to interfere with daily life and functioning.

So, are we all destined to decline? No!

A major misconception regarding the human adult brain has been that it is unable to change—that aging results in a gradual, unavoidable and irreversible decline of cognitive abilities. Many also wrongly believe that major neurocognitive disorder, or what is commonly referred to as "dementia," is a normal part of aging. Contemporary research, however, has shown that far from being unable to change, the brain actually exhibits neuroplasticity, or the ability to adapt based on experience and environmental influences. Each day, there is new, exciting research about the various ways that the brain can reorganize structures and functions. A good example of this comes from research with people who have had strokes or traumatic brain injuries. Through rehabilitation, they are able to regain functioning that appeared to be lost. Neuroplasticity not only refers to these dramatic changes, but also to the subtle changes that take place with everyday living, such as those produced by the consumption of certain brain-healthy foods (e.g., cold water fish that provide omega-3 fatty acids), commitment to an aerobic exercise program (e.g., regular brisk walking), or the pursuit of novel cognitive experiences (e.g., learning to speak a new language). Thus, many of our behaviors have the potential to change our brains and improve our cognitive functioning at any age.

What exactly does "cognitive functioning" include?

In this chapter, we will first review what is meant by the broad term "cognitive functioning" and then we will consider one of the most commonly recognized aging-related deviations from healthy cognitive functioning: dementia. The remainder of the book will address ways of protecting and maintaining brain health throughout the lifespan.

Cognitive Functions

Cognitive functioning is a broad term used to describe the mental processes related to generating new and using existing knowledge, such as memory, attention, judgment, reasoning, comprehension and problem-solving. We will summarize the major cognitive domains below. We will be referring to many different brain regions as a primer to the brain – do not get bogged down by the details. Rather, try to appreciate how complex and fascinating cognitive functioning is.

Memory

Memory is an extremely complex process, but we typically do not give it much conscious thought until it starts to fail us. Memory involves attending to a particular set of stimuli, interpreting the stimuli and filing the different components (emotions, sights, sounds, etc.) in different parts of the brain. When we want to recall something, we have to retrieve these various components and integrate them. Retrieved memories may differ a bit each time as a function of new information, learning, perceptions and other factors. A structure called the hippocampus is largely responsible for this integration of information (we'll be talking about the hippocampus a lot, so here's a memory aid often used by medical students to remember the importance of the region: imagine a hippo on campus directing traffic).

There are various types of memory that involve many parts of the brain. Thus, it's not uncommon for people to have a problem with one type of memory but not with others.

Working Memory. Working memory is crucial for everyday functioning. Also called short-term memory (STM), working memory can be thought of as a container where information is housed for retrieval a short time later – it holds information while we focus our attention on other tasks and behaviors. So, if you are in the kitchen and decide you want to get your green sweater from your bedroom before you leave the house, that piece of information is put in the STM container. Along the way to the bedroom you may start thinking about other things and then when you get to the closet you have to retrieve the information about the green sweater from that container.

As you age, there may be times when you get to the closet and the STM is empty! The container can be "leaky," such that crucial information is forgotten, leaving you bemused as to why you are even standing at the closet in the first place. Occasional, minor memory lapses (e.g., forgetting why you walked into the kitchen, where you put your glasses or where you left your keys, etc.) can be a normal consequence of age-related changes in the brain. It is when these lapses become more frequent and interfere with daily functioning that an underlying condition may be the cause.

Long-term Memory. Long-term memory is intended for the storage of information over an extended period of time. Long-term memory can be divided into two subcategories: explicit (i.e., declarative) memory and implicit (i.e., procedural) memory. One way to think about these distinctions is that explicit memories require conscious effort to recall, while implicit memories do not.

Explicit Memory
Declarative Memory. Declarative memory is the deliberate recall of information that can be stated as words. Declarative memory is mediated by the left temporal lobe, a location also associated with language processing. There are two forms of declarative memory:

> *Episodic Memory.* Episodic memory is the recall of autobiographical events and personal experiences. So, if your partner is reminiscing about a vacation you took together a few years ago and you have no recollection of it at all, this is an episodic memory failure. The decline of episodic memory is often readily apparent to loved ones as individuals forget the details of important past experiences. Some episodic memory processing occurs in the left temporal lobe.

Semantic Memory. Semantic memory is the recall of meanings, understandings and other factual information. Trying to remember the date of a certain historical event is a semantic memory exercise. Being unable to recall someone's name is a commonly reported semantic memory failure.

Implicit Memory

Procedural Memory. Procedural memory is the unconscious recall of how to do various tasks and how to perform skills. For example, when you ride a bike you are using procedural memory in that, for the most part, it is done on "auto-pilot"; you do not have to think about pedaling. Initially, the learning of skills is explicit as you consciously plan and focus on doing an action. But with practice, this becomes implicit. Anatomical structures associated with procedural memory processing include the striatum, basal ganglia and cerebellum, among other areas.

Attention

Attention directs consciousness, highlighting different parts of the world. Sometimes, this is overt—a conscious, intentional process—but other times the process is less obvious—it can seem like something (or someone) literally "grabs" our attention. There are several different types of attention:

Focused attention involves narrowing your attention to a very specific auditory, visual or tactile stimulus. For example, a runner waiting for the starter's gun to go off may hone her attention so keenly on the starter that she may not even notice the crowd or other runners.

Sustained attention is the ability to maintain attention on one object or activity for a continuous period of time. This is more difficult than most people imagine. One way to assess sustained attention is to have a subject watch a computer screen as different stimuli, for example letters of the alphabet, are presented and to hit the spacebar when he or she sees a certain letter. This test typically goes on for five minutes and most people experience difficulty maintaining the desired behavioral response for the duration of the task. Children with Attention Deficit Disorder (ADD) are often yawning, stretching and looking around the room after about only forty seconds!

Selective attention is similar to sustained attention but involves the ability to resist shifting focus in the face of distracting or competing stimuli.

Alternating attention requires shifting focus from one stimulus to another in the course of one activity. For example, playing sports often involves surveying action from different parts of the court or field to determine your next move.

Divided attention, better known as multi-tasking, involves switching your attention between two or more unrelated activities. The brain can actually only fully focus on one thing at a time so multi-tasking is really task switching.

Although the frontal lobe is the main region associated with attention, many areas of the brain from the visual to the spatial areas are involved. Treatment for ADD targets stimulation of the frontal lobe, since under-stimulation can lead to attention difficulties.

Executive Functioning

Executive functioning is the ability to plan and execute actions. An action can be as simple as going to fetch something from another room, which requires making the decision, planning how to do it, paying attention, initiating the movement and keeping the goal in mind, among other processes. This is yet another example of integrated action, which is mediated in various parts of the frontal lobe. A failure of any one of these steps (e.g., a working memory deficit) can impact the ability to successfully execute the action.

Visual-Spatial Processing

Orienting ourselves in space requires processing incoming sensory information as well as executing motor movements. The occipital areas at the back of the brain are largely responsible for visual processing and the parietal lobes are the primary areas for spatial orientation and awareness. The sensory-motor strip in the central area of the brain coordinates incoming information with the planning and execution of motor movement.

Language and Speech

There are several areas of the brain involved in language comprehension and speech production. Wernicke's area in the upper temporal lobe is where words are processed and also where they are selected for speech. Broca's area in the frontal lobe is responsible for speech production and meaning, while Geschwind's territory in the front of the parietal lobe integrates sensory and physical sensations, helping to match the right words to thoughts.

There are several different types of speech and language problems that can occur with various cognitive disorders:

Global Aphasia refers to general deficits in comprehension, naming and speech production.

Production Aphasia is the inability to articulate words or string them together.

Conduction Aphasia involves the substitution of sounds and speech errors, where comprehension and fluency are retained.

Transcortical Sensory Aphasia is the inability to comprehend, name, read, or write, despite the fact that learned material can be readily recalled.

Transcortical Motor Aphasia manifests as non-fluent speech where comprehension is retained.

Sensory Aphasia is the inability to understand language along with general comprehension difficulties.

Social Cognition

Effective social interaction requires the ability to accurately interpret what others are thinking and feeling such that one can respond or react appropriately. Various parts of the brain are involved in these processes. In the frontal areas of the brain, there is a system of interconnecting neurons called the mirror neuron system, which some suggest is responsible for the ability to empathize. This process also involves being able to "read" facial and non-verbal expressions.

Emotion

The physiology of emotion is linked to arousal of the nervous system. The brain's main goal is survival and the fight-or-flight response can be activated in about one-twelfth of a second following the perception of a threat. An area of the brain called the limbic system includes critical structures, such as the amygdala, that monitor all incoming stimuli for potential harm and signal other areas of the brain in response to a potential threat. Many researchers believe that this process is the basis of fear and anxiety. The limbic system connects with the frontal lobe, which analyzes the information and can inhibit an emotional response. Frontal lobe damage often results in less inhibition, leading to impulsivity and the inappropriate acting out of emotions. Sometimes, sudden changes in personality can be attributed to frontal lobe dysfunction.

The fight-or-flight response creates a heightened state of arousal, which feels like fear. The stress response is designed to maximize energy production and output so that we can fight or run in order to defend ourselves. However, the flip side of this response is energy conservation as the body tries to recoup and recover. The energy conservation phase can seem a lot like depression, with little motivation for action, withdrawal and excessive sleep.

It may seem that with all of these various parts and functions, it is inevitable that something will "go wrong."

Indeed, as suggested by the complexity of the cognitive system, a deficit in any of the aforementioned structures can lead to noticeable and perhaps debilitating losses of function. However, we also know that the brain can adapt and restructure in order to maintain functioning.

Despite what the scientific community once thought about the brain's inability to create new neural pathways beyond childhood, we now know that we can not only create new connections but also brain cells throughout the lifespan through a process called neurogenesis. Keeping new cells alive and preserving function through remapping of the brain are challenges and, as you will learn later in this book, key goals of a new program in brain health called the Cognitive Therapeutics Method™.

The brain is an interconnected network that operates as an integrated whole. While it is true that certain functions, such as language, are generally "housed" in certain areas of the brain, it is too simplistic to think of the brain as a collection of bounded, compartmentalized areas. Moreover, the brain has the ability to adapt and relocate functions from one area to another based on experience. This awe-inspiring process is called neuroplasticity, or cortical remapping. This process is beautifully illustrated through the famous case of Daniel Kish, who was blinded when he was only one year old. Daniel, by making clicking sounds with his tongue and attuning himself to the echoes he heard in response, taught himself the skill of echolocation. Yes, that's right—Daniel used the same process that bats and dolphins use to navigate the world. This is an example of an adaptation made possible through neuroplasticity.

Normally the occipital areas of the brain responsible for processing vision are dormant in blind people. But, when Daniel's brain was studied it showed that the visual areas of his brain had connected with the auditory areas enabling him to "see" sounds. Essentially, his brain had reallocated unused connections in order to accommodate a new skill. In case you think this is a fluke, scientists have found many other cases of individuals compensating for the loss of one sensory modality (e.g., blindness) by using another sense. The brain truly has a great capacity to adapt and reorganize itself. Harnessing the power of neuroplasticity is at the heart of the Cognitive Therapeutics Method™ and other advances in maintaining cognitive functioning.

Cognitive Therapeutics

Developed by Home Care Assistance, the Cognitive Therapeutics Method™ is an activities-based cognitive stimulation program designed to keep individuals mentally sharp. Based on a comprehensive literature review of non-pharmacological approaches to delay the onset of neurocognitive disorders and slow the progression of cognitive decline, the Method involves hundreds of activities that engage all areas of cognitive functioning. Like a workout for your brain, the program is designed for everyone – from those who are cognitively healthy and want to maintain their mental acuity to those with deficits in cognitive functioning that are interfering with quality of life.

10

Researchers have become increasingly interested in neuroplasticity in recent decades given the many conditions that result in the gradual loss of neurons. While the brain does tend to slow down with age and some functions may be compromised (e.g., reaction time), it is important to remember that aging itself is not a disease. Serious cognitive decline, while more common with increasing age, is the result of an underlying neurodegenerative disease.

What are these neurodegenerative diseases?

Some of the more common diseases and conditions contributing to declines in cognitive functioning are described below.

Dementia

Dementia, also called major neurocognitive disorder, is a general term used to describe a decline in mental abilities severe enough to interfere with daily functioning. There are many causes of dementia, such as Alzheimer's disease and Parkinson's disease, with quite different manifestations. We will review some of these below:

Alzheimer's Disease

Alzheimer's is the most common cause of dementia, accounting for between 60 and 80% of cases. It is the sixth leading cause of death in the United States, the seventh leading cause of death in Canada and the third leading cause of death in Australia. In addition to genetic factors, a variety of lifestyle factors (e.g., head trauma, obesity) have been linked with an increased risk of Alzheimer's.

There is an ongoing debate about how early Alzheimer's can be detected. It is a progressive disease and is often divided into early, middle and late stages. The typical time frame from detection to late stage is about eight years.

Initially, deficits in working and declarative memory are evident. In this early phase people can't hold information in the short-term memory buffer container. They may often forget people's names and why they entered the kitchen, for example. Such memory failures are not uncommon with aging. However, the frequency of their occurrence is the important factor to consider. Also, there is a difference between going into a room, forgetting why you are there and then remembering, and not being able to recall the purpose at all, even when prompted with cues.

As the disease progresses, visual-spatial processing also becomes impaired, increasing the likelihood of balance problems and falls. This can have the secondary effect of reducing a person's confidence in his or her mobility, resulting in less activity and isolation. Reduced motor function can result in incontinence, speech difficulties and even problems with the ability to swallow. In the later stages, many cognitive functions are compromised. Executive function is severely impacted, as it depends on effective coordination of many parts of the brain. Because cognitive functioning and neurological capacity in general are severely impacted, anxiety, anger, fear and depression are not uncommon.

Vascular Dementia (VaD)

Vascular dementia is caused by diseases that disrupt blood flow to the brain. Blockages anywhere in the system that supplies blood to the brain can lead to damage or death of many important parts of the brain's machinery. Vascular dementia is the second most common form of dementia, in part because of the incidence of cardiovascular disease in the senior population. The disease duration is typically five years.

A cerebrovascular accident (CVA), or stroke, is the most common cause of VaD. There are ischemic strokes, where a clot blocks blood flow to an area of the brain, and hemorrhagic strokes, where bleeding occurs inside or around brain tissue. These events deprive various areas of the brain of oxygen, resulting in tissue damage or death. A third of people who suffer recurrent strokes are likely to develop dementia.

Although those with VaD can present with a variety of cognitive impairments, the most common initial deficit is in executive functioning. Decline of frontal lobe functioning results in inabilities to plan, monitor and execute tasks. Initially at least, memory disturbance is not markedly noticeable.

Frontotemporal Dementia (FTLD)

Frontotemporal dementia, as its name suggests, impacts the frontal and temporal areas, and thus is characterized by behavioral and language deficits. Because this condition affects the frontal lobe, sudden changes in personality and social behavior are not uncommon. The course of this disease typically runs from two to ten years with progressive cognitive deterioration eventually necessitating around-the-clock care.

Genetic correlates of variations of FTLD have been found. For example, Pick's Disease, a form of FTLD, is caused by the aggregation of tau proteins in neurons. As the disease progresses, it impacts speech production and other cognitive faculties to varying degrees—some people become mute, some retain speech capability but comprehension fails, some become unable to recognize faces and some develop Parkinsonism-type symptoms like muscle rigidity and tremors. Deficits in social perception and emotional processing are common to all variants of FTLD.

Parkinson's Disease (PD) and Lewy Body Dementia (LBD)
Parkinson's disease is a chronic, degenerative condition.
Although most people recognize the condition for its muscle
and motor dysfunctions, it also has associated cognitive
deficits. The disease is characterized by the loss of dopamine-
generating cells. As a neurotransmitter, dopamine is involved
in motor control, reward, motivation, pleasure, behavioral
choice and immune system function. Round, compact masses
of proteins known as Lewy bodies are also a marker of the
disease when found in an area of the brain called the
substantia nigra, the hub of dopamine production.

There's no exact agreement on how PD and LBD differ, but
one very general guideline is that if motor deficits precede
cognitive problems, PD is diagnosed and when it's the other
way around, LBD is diagnosed. Cognitive symptoms
associated with LBD include attentional, executive function
and visual-spatial deficits, hallucinations, and even loss of
consciousness.

Apart from characteristic tremors and movement difficulties
(which many people with PD do not exhibit), those with PD
can also suffer from executive function, mood and memory
problems. Given the difficulties with the initiation of
movement it is no surprise that procedural memory and
learning are also impacted as well as other more subtle
motor movements, like speech production. As the disease
progresses, loss of confidence in mobility can lead to
withdrawal and isolation.

Mixed Dementia (MD)
Mixed dementia is the term given to overlapping and
co-occurring forms of dementia mentioned above. It is unclear
whether MD is a diagnosis in itself or simply two or more

dementias occurring at the same time. How co-occurring dementias impact each other is a matter for further research. For example, Alzheimer's and Vascular dementia often occur together, though how they interact and impact each other remains to be seen.

Multiple Sclerosis (MS)

Multiple sclerosis is a disorder that affects the myelin sheath, the protective cover on neurons. Myelin is critical for effective communication between neurons. Poor myelination at birth is associated with factors like malnourishment, maternal drug use and stress, and manifests as serious cognitive problems and developmental delays in children. Because lesions in MS can be localized, symptoms vary in type and intensity. Difficulties in attention, executive function, working memory, procedural learning, processing speed and social perception have all been found in people with MS. Often, multiple processes are impacted by the disease.

MS can be an intermittent, relapsing condition in which sufferers go through spells of flare-ups which then remediate, or it can be a progressive condition in which there is a general deterioration over time. According to a 2008 World Health Organization report, MS is the leading cause of disability in middle-aged adults.

But how do you know if these conditions or deficits are present —how can you "measure" dementia?

Having outlined fundamental cognitive functions and dementia, we'll know explore one component of disease diagnosis – how brain activity and functioning are assessed.

Brain Imaging

Brain imaging, often in the form of magnetic resonance imaging (MRI), positron emission tomography (PET) or single photon emission computed tomography (SPECT) scans, involves taking a photo of the brain to determine whether there are structural or other noticeable abnormalities. There are variations on these procedures. For example, a functional MRI (fMRI) shows where activity occurs, or does not occur, in the brain while it is performing cognitive tasks. The fMRI has been instrumental in the explosion of cognitive research in the past decade, as researchers look to see what areas of the brain become active during different tasks and situations.

Images are typically compared against a database of people matched for age and gender. For example, a NeuroQuant is an image of the hippocampus, the area of the brain responsible for integrating memory. You can assess how "normal" or "not normal" an individual's hippocampus is by comparing his or her NeuroQuant to normative database results.

Brainwaves

The electroencephalography (EEG) and the quantitative EEG (QEEG) look at brainwave activity at different sites in the brain to determine variables such as the type and amount of activity, and the interconnectedness of the left and right brain hemispheres. To provide a simplified overview, there are four main brainwaves with different electrical frequencies as shown in the box below. Like brain imaging, EEG and QEEG data are compared against a normative database to establish whether observed patterns are within normal parameters or not. There has been much research that shows the characteristic footprints of many brain conditions. For example, anxiety often shows up as high levels of Beta wave activity in the right hemisphere. Such findings can, therefore, aid in the diagnosis of psychiatric, cognitive and neurological problems.

Four Main Brainwaves		
Delta	1-4 Hz	Sleep state, deep sleep
Theta	4-8 Hz	Drowsiness, deep meditation
Alpha	9-13 Hz	Relaxed wakefulness
Beta	13-30 Hz	Information processing, anxiety

Cognitive Testing

An important component of assessing and diagnosing dementia is through cognitive testing, often conducted by a neuropsychologist. There are myriad tests that assess the gamut of cognitive functions. Some of these are general in nature and provide an overall score based on subtests of different abilities (e.g., Wechsler Intelligence test), while others are very specific (e.g., The Test of Variable Attention, also called the TOVA). All good tests are standardized against a normative database, matched by age, gender and other demographic variables. Thus, individuals are provided scores of how their functioning measures up against others similar to them.

Medical Tests

There are many tests of physical functions that are helpful in diagnosing dementia. For example, measures of insulin and blood-glucose can determine risks associated with cardiovascular disease, blood flow and glucose availability, all important variables in brain health.

Today, genetic testing is more readily available and can tell a lot about a person's predisposition for specific neurocognitive disorders or other conditions. Note, however, that a genetic predisposition to a disease (e.g., possessing the APOE e4 gene appears to increase the risk for Alzheimer's disease) doesn't mean that a person definitively will get the disorder, just as the lack of a genetic predisposition doesn't equate to zero risk of one day developing the disorder.

All of these tests are sources of information that should be used alongside the person's self-report and, observation by both professionals and others to create an integrated picture of brain function.

Now, having briefly considered the brain, its functions and how different forms of dementia can cause cognitive impairments, let us explore some of treatments designed to preserve and even boost brain function. As you read on you will see that in addition to formal treatments, there are many behaviors linked to brain health, including diet, exercise, mental stimulation, and socialization. Adopting a brain-healthy lifestyle is one of the best ways to support optimal cognitive function.

CHAPTER 2
TREATMENTS FOR DEMENTIA: PHARMACOLOGICAL AND BEYOND

Much public attention around the globe has turned to efforts to find effective treatments for one of the greatest health challenges of the 21st century: dementia. A recent study found that for each person diagnosed with dementia, several other individuals suffer from undiagnosed cognitive impairments that negatively impact their quality of life. This speaks to the overwhelming societal cost and burden of cognitive decline and the associated need for more effective treatments. Until recently, pharmacological interventions were considered the only treatment for dementia, despite fairly low efficacy. However, exciting new research grounded in neuroplasticity suggests that other techniques can change the brain in remarkable ways. In this chapter we will review the pharmacological approaches to dementia and then consider the brave, innovative and exciting world of neuroplasticity.

Pharmacological Treatments
Most forms of dementia are degenerative, meaning that they cannot be cured, and progressive, meaning that they worsen over time. Like many irreversible diseases, treatment primarily has been oriented towards effectively managing the condition and providing the best quality of life for as long as possible.

Pharmacological treatments are used:

- To slow the progression of the disease
- To manage the symptoms of the disease
- To manage co-occurring conditions (e.g., depression)

Despite the many research dollars that have gone into trying to demonstrate the ability of pharmaceutical treatments to reverse symptoms or significantly slow disease progression, primarily in Alzheimer's disease, the results have not been promising.

Pharmacological Treatments to Slow the Progression of Disease
Despite the lack of long-term efficacy, a review of the primary mechanisms underlying Alzheimer's disease allows us to understand the targets of many of the presently available medications.

In Alzheimer's disease, a combination of factors leads to the formation of tangles and plaques that kill neurons and/or significantly inhibit their functioning by reducing their ability to communicate with other neurons. To date, medications designed to prevent the formation of plaques have not been successful.

Another implicated mechanism is the death of cells that release acetylcholine (ACh). This neurotransmitter is important for many functions including muscle movement, urinary and GI tract function, learning and memory formation. In theory, anything that would increase the availability of ACh should improve the communication and functioning of brain cells. Cholinesterase inhibitors are designed to do just that by temporarily preventing the breakdown of ACh by the enzyme cholinesterase. Though cholinesterase inhibitors have primarily been tested in the treatment of Alzheimer's disease, they may also be effective for the treatment of Lewy Body dementia, vascular dementia and mixed dementia, as data suggest that ACh depletion may play a role in those conditions as well.

Cholinesterase inhibitors on the market include Donepezil (Aricept), Rivastigmine (Exelon) and Galantamine (Razadyne). While Aricept is approved to treat all stages of dementia, the other cholinesterase inhibitors are approved only for the treatment of early to middle stages of the condition. Studies show that people who benefit from these medications can expect to see the progression of the disease slowed for about six months to a year. Some of the side effects of these drugs include nausea, vomiting, weight loss, loss of appetite and diarrhea, as well as an increased risk of falls, an important consideration as falls are a leading cause of injuries in the senior population.

Memantine (Namenda) is the second type of pharmacological treatment on the market. This drug works to reduce the amount of glutamate, a neurotransmitter than has excitatory effects, in the brain. Similar to Aricept, Namenda has been shown to produce modest effects in those suffering from moderate to severe Alzheimer's. There is some evidence of improved results in those who take both Aricept and Namenda, but it is still too early to know the clinical significance of the combination therapy and long-term outcomes.

Pharmacological Treatments to Manage the Symptoms of Disease and Co-occurring Conditions
In addition to medications designed to improve cognitive functioning or slow the disease process, many people with dementia are also prescribed drugs to treat associated, non-cognitive conditions. For example, those with vascular dementia are often treated with medications designed to combat hypertension, diabetes and high cholesterol, and some people with Parkinson's are given Levodopa (Sinemet) to better manage physical symptoms.

It is common for adults with dementia to also have psychiatric comorbidities, such as a depression or anxiety. In fact, the presence of these conditions can often complicate diagnosis of dementia, because depression and dementia manifest similarly in older adults.

Harnessing Neuroplasticity with Non-Pharmacological Treatments

Given the limited efficacy of medications in making a significant impact on disease progression, many researchers have turned to non-pharmacological interventions, such as cognitive therapy. In order to understand how cognitive stimulation may help slow cognitive decline, we'll start by considering one of the most exciting developments in neuroscience – the notion that the brain is actually incredibly adaptable.

As we mentioned in the first chapter, neuroplasticity refers to the brain's ability to reorganize neural connections, create new connections and, in some cases, create new neurons. In general, neuroplasticity can occur for two reasons: as a result of learning and experience or as a result of damage to the brain.

While researchers previously believed that the process of neurogenesis stopped shortly after birth, it is now generally accepted that new brain cells can be formed throughout the lifespan. Indeed, neurogenesis actually happens all

Physical Adaptation

Our bodies adapt to the environment and show signs of plasticity, too. For example, people living in far Northern Canada hunt seals and whales for food. They fish in ice-cold polar water. If someone from California were to try to fish in the same polar waters, he or she would probably experience unpleasant consequences such as hand cramping. The hands of the natives actually stay warm in the icy water! That's adaptation; their bodies adapted to the cold climate by increasing the number of capillaries to get more blood flow to the extremities, especially the hands and fingers. That is the type of adaptation that happens over generations.

the time to replace cells that naturally die or become non-functional. For example, recent research suggests that the annual turnover of cells in the hippocampus, the part of the brain that manages memory, is about 1.75%.

Can neuroplasticity help maintain functioning in Alzheimer's Disease?

Several studies suggest that the answer is "yes." Let us consider how neuroplasticity works and why researchers are excited about this non-pharmacological approach to the treatment of cognitive decline.

Of Mice, Musicians, and Meditators

It can be fascinating to read the studies that come out of the field of neuroscience, not only because of the complexity of the brain but also because of the unique and creative study designs – and subjects – that are often used.

In one study, rats learning a skilled motor task showed more development in the motor areas of the brain than those doing a less skilled task.

Looking at humans, one study showed that the area of the brain associated with fine motor movement of the hand was more developed in those musicians who played stringed instruments. Another study comparing brain responses to tones in amateur and professional musicians as well as those with no musical skills found that the amount of grey matter in the area of the brain associated with processing tones was significantly different among the groups based on the level of musical sophistication. Were the brain differences noted in both of these studies innate or the result of learning? A study comparing the brains of professional keyboard musicians, amateurs and non-musicians ggests that the answer is learning. Like the previous study, professionals had more grey matter in various skill-related areas of the brain and the increased volume was associated with *the amount of time spent practicing.*

Research on neuroplasticity has also been explored in another group of individuals whose brains suggest an association between a learned skill and neural changes: meditators. Cortical thickness typically decreases with age, but in one study seasoned meditators showed less decline in cortical thickness and better performance on an attention test than their non-meditating peers. This observation suggests that meditation may offer some protective effects against aging.

Learning the Streets of London

It is perhaps no surprise, given the complexity of the brain, that neuroscientists are employing some very creative study designs to explore cognitive function across different contexts. A famous study took to the streets of one of the world's great capitals for more proof of the impact of learning on the structure and function of the brain.

Anyone who has ever been to London knows that there is no logic to the names of the myriad, scattered streets. Moreover, as an older city, London was not designed on a grid system or any convenient system at all. So, if you're an aspiring taxi driver in London, you have a lot of learning and memorization to do. There are 25,000 streets within a six-mile radius of Charing Cross Station, a focal point in central London, alone. Training to pass the licensure test typically takes three to four years.

A creative team of neuroscientists decided to explore the structure of the parts of the brain that would be implicated in learning the London streets. Specifically, researchers assessed memory in a group of students enrolled in the cab driver education program through MRIs of their hippocampi and formal memory tests. They found that parts of the hippocampus grew over the course of the years of the individuals' training. Moreover, the extent of growth was related to success in the course. Thus, those who performed better experienced greater brain growth than their less successful peers.

This study, like the others mentioned above, creates a roadmap for further research and strongly suggests that behavioral and cognitive practice result in brain changes. Thus, neuroplasticity can occur as a result of learning and experience.

Neuroplasticity can also occur when the brain is injured, presumably for compensatory reasons.

Neuroscientists have to create a map of which parts of the brain are associated with different movements and parts of the body. This is called the "cortical motor map." In clinical cases where the brain is damaged, changes to the "cortical map" have been noted, suggesting that the brain has the capacity to relocate motor functions from a damaged area to a non-damaged one.

An elegant demonstration of the relocation of function after injury can be found in a study on adult squirrel monkeys that had lesions in an area of the brain related to hand movements. After retraining the monkeys, their cortical maps reflected that changes had occurred. In some cases, hand movements seemed to be associated with areas on the cortical map that were previously associated with shoulder and elbow movements.

One question is how the intensity and frequency of rehabilitation exercises influence neuroplasticity and changes in the cortical motor map. Edwin Taub developed an extreme form of rehabilitation for upper extremity injuries. His treatment focused on frequent and intense use of the affected limb, often for several hours a day. Never has the phrase "use it or lose it" been more appropriate.

These more extreme rehabilitative measures were associated with improved use and ability of the affected limb. In addition, imaging studies suggested that the degree of cortical reorganization that occurred was proportional to the amount of use of the affected part of the body. Thus, the brain can, and often does, respond to challenge.

If the brain can reallocate its resources naturally, the question then becomes whether it can be helped in its efforts by other interventions.

For example, could drugs or non-pharmacological, cognitive exercises help the brain reorganize itself? Some studies have shown that stimulants can facilitate the recovery of cognitive function in people with brain injuries and tumors. The proper use of medications along with progressively challenging rehabilitation exercises, have also been shown to enhance the rehabilitation process. It is the non-pharmacological approaches, however, that are garnering the most interest and showing the most potential.

As you will learn in subsequent chapters, lifestyle factors, such as nutrition, exercise and stress can also impact the brain's ability to adapt. It appears that in order for the new cells created by neurogenesis to survive, they need to be exercised by keeping the mind engaged—that means challenging the brain, learning new information and new skills. Physical movement seems to also be important for cognitive change. One study showed that aerobic exercise seemed to have the greatest effect on the frontal areas of the brain and the hippocampus, areas that affect memory, planning and judgment.

So while neuroplasticity holds great promise, it is not a simple, one-size-fits-all process. It is subject to influence by a variety of factors. Nonetheless, the brain and the nervous system's ability to modify both structure and function suggests that neuroplasticity is one path to the management, prevention and possibly successful treatment of neurodegenerative diseases.

We'll now consider how various behaviors can be used to preserve or even improve brain function.

CHAPTER 3
SOCIAL ACTIVITY AND THE BRAIN

Over the past two decades, there has been considerable attention focused on the impact of social activity on wellbeing. Generally, the research suggests that being sociable is good for your health. Studies show that more isolated people have worse health and typically higher risks of mortality. Indeed, it has been observed that there is a higher risk of mortality after the loss of a spouse – referred to as the "bereavement effect." Further speaking to link between socialization and wellbeing, the risk is mitigated when the surviving spouse has greater social support.

When people hear about the positive effects of social activity, most think back to highly memorable or exciting shared events. As great as those experiences are, socialization doesn't necessarily have to involve peaks of emotion or significant events to produce beneficial effects. Even simple, day-to-day interactions with others can have positive effects on wellbeing.

Let's meet Jane.

Consider a scenario involving a woman named Jane who is invited over to her neighbor Nancy's (memory aid: N for neighbor) house for some coffee and conversation.

Jane's brain will start to be engaged even before stepping foot inside Nancy's house! She will anticipate the situation; she will probably think about what is going to happen, especially in this case as she knows that one of the neighbor's friends, Franny (memory aid: F for friend), will also be there. She has to consider what to wear and her general appearance. She may visualize what will happen.

Jane arrives at her neighbor's and is greeted by Nancy and Franny, with whom she is only minimally acquainted. All sorts of cognitive processes are involved at this point. Yes, the introductions at some level are what are called "reflexive language" — the niceties of small talk exchange, such as "How are you?", "I'm fine," etc. However, they still require attention and judgment (e.g., when to switch out of that into something more substantive).

The initial interaction immediately activates memory. "Didn't we meet before?" asks Franny. Jane has to scan her memory bank. She has a recollection of a past social gathering but is not sure whether the memory is accurate and has to make a judgment about volunteering it into the conversation. She thinks about saying it and rehearses it mentally before speaking.

"Wasn't it at Don Smith's retirement party?" Jane suggests. Now Jane is scanning Franny's face for signs of recognition. The part of the brain that interprets faces and gestures kicks into gear as Jane waits to find out whether her memory is accurate.

"Yes, that's right!" says Franny enthusiastically. Jane's brain now processes the feedback and she experiences an emotional lift on account of the fact that her memory was indeed accurate and Franny produced a positive response. Neurotransmitters are released and neurons start communicating with each other in the emotional areas of the brain.

"Let us sit down," says Nancy, motioning her two guests into the living room.

As they walk to take their seats, Nancy says something to Franny about Don Smith's children.

The conversation seems to have moved from small talk to something more substantial and Jane now studies Franny intently. She is processing Franny's body language and facial expressions. She is paying very close attention to her words, especially speech rhythm, tone and a host of other factors related to listening. As she processes what Franny is saying (and not saying directly), Jane's frontal lobe assesses and judges the content, possibly matching it up to memories. Jane doesn't necessarily have to consciously will these things to happen for them to occur.

The three women are still standing, stopped by the living room seating arrangement.

Having processed the interaction between her neighbor and the friend, Jane now thinks about making a comment. This requires numerous cognitive operations. Attention circuits are involved, as Jane has to attend to what she is saying (I know some people do not seem ever to think about what they are saying but from a neurocognitive perspective, most people do). She also has to pay attention to the reactions of the other two women, again perceiving and making judgments about their responses.

As evidenced by the example above, speech is a complex process even though it may seem so automatic for most of us. Not only do you have to determine what you want to convey but you also have to choose words, tone, rhythm, pattern and gestures, while at the same time monitoring yourself and your audience. The audio-vocal or audiological loop involves a complex neurological interaction, which amounts to a good brain workout.

It is now time for the ladies to sit down. Jane has to look at the seating arrangements and determine where to sit based on perceptions of Nancy, Franny, their relationships and a variety of other factors. For example, if she sits in the farthest chair and the other two take seats closer together, will she be on the outside or appear aloof?

Eventually, the other two take their seats and Jane chooses one that is well-placed to allow her equal access to the two ladies.

Jane has been at her neighbor's for less than three minutes. During this short time, her brain has been performing a number of complex operations. She has had to use short-term memory (e.g., what did Franny just say?) and a episodic memory (e.g., where did I meet Franny?). She has had to interpret facial expressions and bodily gestures and make judgments about what she has seen and heard. She has had to decide on courses of action and she has had to decide to speak. She has used critical senses and interpreted a lot of sensory information. She has had to make social judgments, like where to sit. She has experienced emotional responses. She has had to adapt to the changing and evolving circumstances of the interaction. This simple interaction has thus far provided Jane with a neurocognitive workout of sorts.

As their time together goes on, Jane enjoys the conversation and the company of her two friends. Her brain continues to perform the many operations required in social interaction, what is technically called "social cognition." Now, she is feeling connected.

The conversation gradually reaches the subject of siblings. Nancy volunteers that her sister, now deceased, felt a lifetime of guilt over miscarrying a child. Despite being assured that this was a medical issue, the sister felt somehow responsible for the loss of the fetus.

When Jane hears this, her eyes start to water. Her emotional change is obvious to the other two women. Nancy is immediately concerned that she has inadvertently stepped on an emotional landmine. There is a pause.

"I've never told anyone this," says Jane. "The same thing happened to me when I was 22. Even though I was told that it could not have been prevented, I've always felt a burden of guilt, as if there was something that I did wrong," Jane softly says, reaching for a tissue as the others watch empathically.

What is empathy? How did Jane feel after sharing something so private?

Empathy

Think back to a really great conversation you had with someone. You seem to be connecting well. The talk seems effortless (even though it is not — see above. The conversation might not be taxing emotionally but still requires a lot of brain activity). When you leave that conversation, how do you feel? Chances are that following a great conversation you feel energized. You might even have a smile on your face.

Now think back to a more negative conversation. You are talking with someone who is moaning about the unfairness of life and complaining about other people's deficiencies and weaknesses. When you leave that conversation, how do you feel? Chances are that you feel drained and down. Here's the thing: you might agree with the substance of what that person is saying but nonetheless listening to complaints can be depressing. Now, you might also be frustrated about this person's flight into victimhood, in which case you'll feel depressed and angry.

One of the more interesting advances in neuroscience has been the discovery of the infrastructure of empathy. Mirror neurons were first described in macaque monkeys and then, humans. Research suggests what we know already: people vary in their capacities to feel empathy. Some people are quite empathic and seem to be able to relate to almost every living thing's perceived mental state, while others can hardly relate to even those closest to them. Studies using brainwave measurements like the EEG have suggested that the mirror neuron circuitry is dysfunctional in people with autism spectrum disorder, a condition characterized by poor social perception and communication, among other deficits.

An interesting fact about mirror neurons is that they allow humans, as well as other animals, to relate at a physical and emotional level. For example, studies show that when a primate sees, for example, an experimenter lifting his arm, the areas of the brain involved in lifting the arm are activated in the primate, too. Hence the "mirror" in mirror neurons. This ability of the brain to model others' behaviors and feel their emotions is a critical aspect of social interaction and a basis of morality.

There have been numerous experiments with primates and other species, which seem to demonstrate that a variety of animals also have what humans would call empathy. Many an animal lover and dog owner will swear that their pets respond to their emotional states, implying that these animals somehow know what a human is feeling.

A 2007 Time magazine article on this subject reported the following story:

> "Russian primatologist Nadia Kohts, who studied nonhuman cognition in the first half of the 20th century, raised a young chimpanzee in her home. When the chimp would make his

way to the roof of the house, ordinary strategies for bringing him down—calling, scolding, offers of food—would rarely work. But if Kohts sat down and pretended to cry, the chimp would go to her immediately. 'He runs around me as if looking for the offender,' she wrote. 'He tenderly takes my chin in his palm... as if trying to understand what is happening.'"

Sometimes such stories make the worldwide news. In 1996, people around the world heard about Binti Jua, the gorilla who tenderly nurtured a toddler who had fallen into her zoo enclosure. She rocked the three-year-old gently in her arms and carried him to the zoo staff.

Social Support

Dr. James Pennebaker has had a distinguished career as a psychologist researching what happens when people do and do not vent. The answer is fairly clear. When people hold their emotions inside and keep them bottled up they tend to have poorer outcomes on a number of health measures. The price of holding emotion inside can be increased muscle tension, decreased mood and increased overall physiological stress levels. Letting that emotion out, for example through a meaningful conversation with a friend, is therapeutic and healthy. Expressive writing has been shown to be helpful in improving mood and overall wellbeing too. Writing your thoughts down or even talking into a tape recorder is still, in part, a social activity in that it involves communication.

As difficult as it is for Jane to share her previously unexpressed emotion, it has some serious health benefits. Talking about her feelings in public converts a painful secret into a shared experience. Nancy and Franny are sympathetic. Instead of the apathetic or critical responses that Jane had imagined for almost fifty years, she hears understanding, empathy and acceptance.

Giving and receiving support are two of the most meaningful human—and non-human—activities (see above). Helping each other is good for the brain as well as the psyche. It wasn't just Jane who had a positive brain experience during her interaction with Nancy and Franny; her two friends benefitted in myriad ways from the exchange as well.

There is the suggestion that what happens in the body during positive social interactions is the opposite of what happens in response to stressful situations. In the fight-or-flight response, barriers go up and the body and mind are geared to fend off attackers, to keep invaders and predators out. Pennebaker and other researchers call this "inhibition." Conversely, positive social interaction really does the opposite; we open up to let people in. Instead of getting physiologically amped up and tense, we become calm and relaxed. Positive social interaction, therefore, can be an antidote to stress.

Back to Jane, Nancy and Franny.

As the afternoon wears on, the three women talk about many different things. They talk, they share, they remember, they laugh, they bond. Jane is shocked when she looks at the clock and realizes that three hours have passed. Normally, she would have had an afternoon nap, but she didn't feel tired at all. (Remember that one benefit of social interaction is that it tends to energize you. Admittedly, there may be people who bore you too, but ideally you can find something meaningful even from those exchanges.)

Reluctantly, the gathering has to break up.

"Jane, would you like to join Franny and me tomorrow morning on our walk?" asks Nancy. "We always go on Wednesdays and we usually walk from here to the lake."

"That would be great," replies Jane as Franny smiles at her. The meeting is set.

The next morning Jane wakes up a little earlier than usual, making sure she is prepared for the morning walk. She knows that she needs to be more active but honestly is not very good about getting herself moving. She walks once in a while but often, when it is time to do some exercise, Jane finds something better to do around the house. Of course, there is not anything better for overall health than exercise — except maybe social interaction.

Good friends can be good influences.

One of the noted values of relationships is that they often encourage people to engage in activities that they wouldn't otherwise do, like exercise. It is sometimes hard to get motivated to exercise on one's own and a solitary workout can also get monotonous. The camaraderie of a group adds another dimension to the exercise, often making it more enjoyable and thus more likely to be repeated. Many older adults who receive care from professional or family caregivers, for example, report physical improvements and boosts in mood when they start engaging in exercise with their caregivers. The caregivers report increased health outcomes as well.

Jane, Nancy and Franny enjoy their walk. It would be difficult to imagine them doing anything healthier as they exercise their bodies and their brains.

As the walk comes to an end, Jane asks the other two women whether they would like to come back to her place for some refreshments. Nancy and Franny gladly accept her invitation.

"I have an idea," says Jane. "Do you girls like to play Scrabble?"
"We do," said Franny, "but you have to know that she is a former English teacher," she says nodding in Nancy's direction.

"Well, I'm a bit of a writer myself," says Jane, getting up to get the Scrabble set.

"Maybe, I won't play," says Franny, "Perhaps I should just watch Clash of the Titans."

Franny does decide to play. The women have a good time exercising their memories, language and attention skills, and judgment.

The women had a very brain-healthy day with exercise, socialization and cognitive stimulation. If they were on their own, they likely would not have gotten this level of variation in brain challenges.

As Nancy and Franny prepare to leave, Jane says, "I had forgotten how nice it is to have company. It's sometimes lonely here, on my own."

"Have you ever thought of getting a dog?" says Franny.

"Thanks a lot!" jokes Nancy, implying that she is now being compared to a four-legged friend.

"I have thought about it, actually," says Jane.

"You know there's research that says having a pet helps lower blood pressure and manage stress. My dog always listens to me and never argues. He's a great companion," says Franny.

Franny is right. Think about it: a dog does provide social interaction. You have to direct attention outward, process information about the dog's behavior, and initiate actions. And of course, walking a dog is a great way to ensure you get exercise. Further, as you have read above, animals aren't stuffed toys; they are sentient, sensitive beings.

Social interaction is stimulating in so many ways – there are the brain processes involved in social cognition and the support and bonding possibilities that have beneficial neurological effects. Social interaction can also be a potent stress reducer and an energizer. Moreover, social interaction is associated with other beneficial activities, such as exercise and cognitive challenges, such as games.

There is some suggestion that aging adults who have larger social networks are healthier and might preserve brain function better than those with smaller networks. Clearly, the more friends you have and the more social circles with which you engage, the more opportunities there are for interaction. It's unclear whether healthier people have more social interactions or more social interactions keep people healthier, but one thing is for sure – having friends and opportunities for social interaction around you is a positive boost to your cognitive health and overall wellbeing.

If socialization is good for the brain can it help those affected by cognitive decline?

There is some debate in the scientific literature about whether social isolation is a consequence of, or contributor to, the symptoms of cognitive decline. Regardless of the direction of the relationship, social interaction in its many different forms clearly leads to more challenge and use of the brain, among other benefits.

As brain function declines, the social possibilities do tend to shrink. Someone in the later stage of Alzheimer's, for example, likely won't be able to hold a very coherent conversation but that doesn't mean efforts to engage a person in this situation should stop. Caregivers should constantly be looking to find new and creative ways to interact with the individual no matter how basic they may seem.

Sometimes, increasing isolation is not a function of neurological decline, but rather mood problems. One of the features of depression is social withdrawal. A critical reason why depression needs to be treated, especially in seniors, is that if left untreated it could lead to loss of social interaction and all the benefits that interacting with our fellow humans—and animals—bestows.

Decreases in social interactions are a common risk with cognitive decline, so social behavior needs to be encouraged and arranged. Here are five things to consider when facilitating social activity:

1. Ensure that the person has all the tools and aids needed to function as well as possible socially. For example, hearing aids can be a necessity. If people are given social opportunities but can't hear a thing, they are likely to be frustrated and more important, discouraged from trying again.

2. Ensure that the social environment is as comfortable and manageable as possible. For example, mobility is a big issue, so easy access to and from social interactions is important. Sufficient lighting will ensure that people can see clearly and stay awake.

3. Match activities to a person's capabilities. While social interaction is helpful, you do not want to overwhelm,

frustrate or depress someone by putting him or her in a situation where he or she feels helpless. If someone does get stressed in a social situation try to determine the cause.

4. Make social interaction as positive as possible. For example, many adults describe pulling away from social interactions with loved ones who can no longer recognize them because this can be a painful and upsetting situation. Instead, take the time to discuss topics they can still remember and stay as positive as possible.

5. Encourage a variety of different types of interactions from different people. Each person brings something unique and that adds variety to every social situation. Being engaged in a number of different social circles— weekly teas with longtime friends, a reading club or a neighborhood walking group—provides diverse and multiple opportunities for continued social engagement.

Social interaction involves a lot of information processing. In the next chapter we will consider how the brain processes information from our senses (and gets another workout by doing so).

CHAPTER 4
SENSORY STIMULATION

Most of us were born with five functioning senses, and this contributed to how fully we were able to engage with and experience the world around us. These senses include hearing, vision, touch, smell and taste. Our senses can change throughout the lifespan for a number of reasons. For example, being exposed to loud noises can cause damage to the ears, resulting in a hearing impairment. Aging itself also brings some predictable changes to our senses (e.g., diminished vision acuity), often making them less able to accurately supply our brain with information about the world around us. Neurodegenerative diseases can also impact sensory processing.

Sensory processing is, like many of the brain's functions, largely unconscious. We hear, see, touch, taste and smell without any concerted effort. In fact, needing to make a conscious effort is often the first sign that the sensory system is not operating as it should.

The sensory system works via receptors at the site of the organ related to a given sense (e.g., a taste receptor on the tongue). These receptors relay information to a nerve center in the spinal cord or elsewhere in the body and then to the brain.

The areas of the brain where sensory information is processed are important in understanding the impacts of different disorders. Not all neurodegenerative disorders affect the same areas of the brain and thus the effects on sensory processing can be quite varied. For example, sound is processed primarily in the temporal lobe, while sight is processed in the occipital lobe. Alzheimer's disease impacts the temporal lobe, suggesting that, in general, sound and hearing are more likely to be affected than sight. On the other hand, Parkinson's disease is associated with damage to more frontal areas of the brain and is, in general, less likely to impact sight and hearing.

Sensory processing can be impacted not only by aging and neurodegenerative diseases, but also by trauma and other health conditions. Decline in sensory processing abilities is typically the result of loss of neurons and connectivity within the brain.

We have seen, however, that the brain can compensate for such changes through neuroplasticity. Research has tried to determine how sensory functioning can be improved or preserved through different techniques. There are various ways of stimulating each of the senses so that they are exercised and remain functional. Sensory stimulation can also aid memory, mood and behavior. In this chapter, we will explore some sensory deficits common with increasing age or the presence of certain neurodegenerative conditions and consider some of the methods that can be used to preserve functioning.

Auditory Stimulation

Decline in auditory processing usually begins when people reach their sixties. Typically, higher frequency processing is affected first, but medium and lower frequency sounds can also become more difficult to process.

Some neurodegenerative conditions affect auditory areas of the brain directly. For example, Alzheimer's disease is associated with changes in the auditory cortex, which leads to problems with verbal encoding and thus recall. This damage can also lead to hallucinations.

The first tactic in trying to improve someone's auditory processing is to make hearing easier through a number of obvious techniques, such as hearing aids. Other ways of presenting sounds, such as slower, more pronounced speech can aid auditory processing. In addition, ensuring there are no other competing voices or ambient noise will also increase the ability of the listener to hear. Repetition can also be helpful for comprehension. Because visual cues like facial and physical gestures are used in communication, looking directly at the person while speaking can also aid processing and comprehension. Similarly, multi-sensorial presentation, where, for example, images are presented along with words, may be more effective than words alone.

Five Ways to Aid Auditory Processing

- Speak slowly and deliberately
- Eliminate other noise
- Look directly at the person
- Use visual aids
- Use repetition

While it is tempting to think that poor hearing primarily impacts social interaction quality, it can also impact memory quality. Memory is the consolidation of a sensory impression so if that impression is garbled or incomplete, the memory will also be affected. We are also much more likely to encode sensory impressions that are already part of our experience. So, for example, interpreting and remembering sounds which represent words we know is much easier than interpreting and remembering sounds with which we have no experience, like words from a different language.

The various sensory components of a memory are stored in different areas of the brain and then recruited by the hippocampus to form coherent recall. This means that a sensory component of a memory has the potential to elicit other aspects of the memory. For example, it's a common experience to hear a song and then be flooded by memories with which the song is associated.

What is the brain-music connection?

As you may know from hearing that song associated with your first kiss or the number one song you played over and over when you were a teenager, music is linked to memories. Even in those experiencing cognitive challenges, music has the potential to elicit already stored memories, such as longer-term and autobiographical details that are so critical in preserving identity.

Marie's mother had been diagnosed with Alzheimer's three years earlier and was now living in an assisted living facility a few miles from Marie's home. Marie made the effort to see her mother on the one day a week she had off from work and on the weekend. She would also call every evening.

Marie was sad to see her mom starting to forget some of the details of her life, and thus began to explore ways of helping to preserve some of those memories. One method she used was photos. Marie framed some photos and put them in prominent positions where her mom would see them, for example by her bed and in the living room.

One of the photos was of her mother and her now deceased father. In it, he was wearing his favorite sweater, which had become something of a family talking point. Marie found a very similar sweater of the same texture and color online and bought it. After giving it to her mother she often found her using it as a cover-up as she sat watching TV or reading.

Marie also made a list of her mother's favorite music and found CDs with many of the songs. She also tracked down DVDs of her mom's favorite TV shows of yesteryear—Lawrence Welk was a particular favorite.

Marie's mom had been a great cook and the family kitchen often was graced with the aroma of freshly baked bread. Occasionally, Marie would simulate that by baking bread or heating it up to create the same aroma when visiting her mom's apartment.

"I think that when mom is cued by these sensory experiences she does have better recall, especially if I prompt her, too," says Marie. "I'm not sure it has improved her memory in the long term but at least it enables her some recollection. And when she is listening to her music or watching her shows, she seems calmer. It's like she is in familiar territory again—at least for a while."

Personally meaningful songs are most effective in triggering memories, promoting calm and stirring connection with others. Talking to the individual and his or her family members might reveal favorite genres or songs associated with important personal events (e.g., a wedding song). In addition, songs from the critical eras of someone's life are likely to be associated with important events.

In addition to stirring memories, personalized music can also provide meaning, a sense of identity and calming familiarity to those with cognitive difficulties. Many studies show that music therapy is associated with decreased agitation and improved mood, cooperation and attention. Music and mood are linked and we all know how the right music can lift our spirits or make us sad. In one study, it was the emotional tone of the music rather than the specific sounds that aided recall in those with Alzheimer's. So, music creates emotions and the emotions themselves can elicit memories.

Singing is another strategy that can help energize us. Apart from saying the Pledge of Allegiance or a prayer in church, typically we do not talk along in unison with other people. Singing, however, adds a social element to vocalization and auditory processing. Singing has been shown to increase participation in various activities for people suffering from cognitive decline and potentially has the ability to aid recall. How many jingles can you recall from TV advertisements? How many are rhymes? There is an area of the brain that is associated with rhythm, stress and intonation of speech, or what technically is called "prosody."

All of the above suggests that music therapy in general can be helpful for those suffering from cognitive decline. In addition, music can activate coordinated movement. In one study Alzheimer's participants responded to music with hand clapping, toe tapping and singing. Live music could also enhance participation as it obviously has more sensory components, not least of which is the sight of the musicians themselves.

Visual Stimulation

As we reach our 40s and 50s, our eyes start to undergo changes that can negatively impact our vision. Many of these potential changes are easy to compensate for and don't have major effects on quality of life, but others can lead to permanent vision loss or blindness. People over 75 are three times more likely to report vision problems than those ages 18-44.

Vision might be predictive of cognitive decline. People with good vision are at least 60% less likely to develop dementia than those with poor vision. However, this could be due to a number of factors related to overall health.

Poor vision might limit a person's ability to engage in social interactions and thus the various benefits that come with these interactions. Poor vision might also limit the willingness or the ability to read, thus cutting off another big source of mental challenge and stimulation. For those in the earlier stages of cognitive decline, poor vision is likely to limit or prevent driving and the sense of independence that comes with being mobile. Poor vision might also impact the ability to exercise on one's own, even going for a walk.

Cognitive decline itself might contribute to visual processing problems by simply making it less likely that people will wear their glasses, or keep up with ophthalmologist appointments.

How does light impact our energy levels?

Exposure to light can be considered a type of visual sensory stimulation. Light is a critical factor in the circadian rhythm, which affects energy and sleep.

From the chart below, you can see that there are times during the day when energy is high and times when it sinks to a low. When energy is high, we are more productive, more able to focus, and more able to cope with problems, people and stress. When energy is low, the reverse is true—we tend to be less focused, more stressed and less able to cope. When energy is low we are also likely to eat more and make less healthy choices. Interestingly enough, the times most associated with bingeing, uncontrolled and often mindless eating of an excessive number of calories, are 4:30 in the afternoon and 10:30 in the evening, when energy is at its lowest.

Typical circadian rhythm pattern for humans

- On waking, energy should be fairly good
- Through the morning hours, energy increases, reaching a peak around midday or soon thereafter
- Energy declines during the afternoon, hitting a low around 4:30 PM
- Energy increases again through the very early evening
- Energy hits another low around 10:30 PM

As we age, there is a shift in the circadian rhythm, so that the peak and low energy times occur earlier in the day. The "early bird special" is actually based on a physiological phenomenon— seniors get hungry earlier because of their shifted circadian rhythms.

Energy is a critical variable for overall health for everybody, but especially seniors. The effective management of energy determines the ability to participate in almost all of the therapeutic activities described in this book. Energy dysregulation has a major impact on several key behaviors.

Poor energy can make a number of healthy behaviors less likely. For example, as mentioned, low energy can encourage unhealthy eating behaviors. Many people think that the afternoon circadian dip is a result of lunch – a "food coma".

While a high glycemic carbohydrate lunch (for example, bread, pasta and soda) can certainly aggravate the dip, it is not the cause of the loss of energy – the circadian rhythm is. You may be tempted to turn to these foods to boost your energy level, but this will only result in a "crash" later. Good nutrition practices such as staying hydrated with water-based drinks, eating protein with plenty of fruits and vegetables and maintaining modest portions can minimize the energy dip. In addition, low energy can make physical activity less likely, thus limiting one of the behaviors that is most critical to brain functioning and health. It can also disrupt the sleep cycle. Deep slow wave sleep is associated with memory consolidation and important restorative brain functions. Napping can interfere with the normal sleep cycle, not only interrupting critical cognitive processes, but also setting off a chain reaction of poor sleep and low energy, perpetuating the cycle.

Low energy can also reduce immune system function, increasing susceptibility to illnesses.

Low energy is associated with lowered mood and depression. In fact, depression can be conceptualized as low energy.

There are ways of managing the low energy times or what are technically called "circadian dips." Taking a brisk walk or doing a similar exercise a couple of hours or so before the afternoon dip occurs can minimize it, or eliminate it altogether. There are other more common ways of dealing with it, of course. In many countries, especially in warmer climates, a siesta is the answer. In other climates like Great Britain, afternoon tea is the solution.

Given that light is an important variable in circadian rhythms, ensuring appropriate exposure at the right times is an important strategy in helping seniors and those experiencing cognitive decline maximize quality of life. If you do not get enough exposure to natural sunlight, one remedy is the use of therapeutic light machines commonly used in the treatment of Seasonal Affective Disorder. There are a variety of delivery systems of the light, from simple lamps to visors. Any use of light therapy in its different forms should take into account personal variations in sleep times and energy levels.

The environment can also be engineered to ensure that lighting levels are appropriately matched to the natural circadian pattern. This would mean bright lights during the day, and much lower illumination just prior to bedtime. Natural light is ideal so open windows in the morning or take a walk outside. Studies focused on this topic suggest that the use of high-intensity ambient lighting throughout the day, especially in the morning, tends to decrease daytime drowsiness and enhance nighttime sleep quality. In another study, the appropriate use of light along with melatonin at night was found to improve nighttime sleep and daytime energy. Melatonin is a natural hormone that regulates the sleep-wake cycle.

What are some common forms of visual stimulation?

The presentation of photos, drawings and personally meaningful images can be used to stimulate memories. Photos of meaningful life events can stimulate episodic memory, in particular. The use of other cues, like music or verbal prompts, can be helpful in eliciting associations with visual presentations.

Art therapy can be considered a form of visual sensory stimulation, although it can also involve other senses providing stimulation to multiple brain areas. For example, some people might prefer to work with clay rather than paint. The handling of the medium of choice, which could be a pencil, paintbrush, chalk, clay or a crayon, involves tactile stimulation and fine motor skills. When done with others, art therapy provides social stimulation, too. Art also provides the opportunity to be creative.

The creative process itself is now getting more attention from neuroscience researchers. You may have heard that creativity comes from the right brain, compared to the left brain, which is supposedly more analytical. This right brain-left brain division is way too simplistic. Creativity involves coordinated action amongst many neural networks. Certain aspects of the creative process seem to involve the temporary relaxation of focused attention in favor of a more intuitive state. On the EEG, this is represented by a reduction of Beta wave activity and an increase in Alpha and Theta waves.

The use of visualization has been shown to be a helpful tool that aids learning and performance. Some studies suggest that when visualizing an action some of the same neural pathways that are employed when actually doing the task are activated. The possibility exists, then, that visualization and the mental rehearsal of skills could be used to improve performance.

Olfactory Stimulation

Human beings can detect at least four thousand different aromas. Our sense of smell is mediated by sensors in the nose which relay information to the olfactory nerve and then to the brain. Separate areas of the brain have different roles in the processing of smell. Currently it is thought that the smell is identified in the piriform cortex and compared with other smell memories in the entorhinal cortex. Interestingly, information from all the other senses passes through a brain structure called the thalamus, which acts like a filtering and relay station. Olfactory information, however, does not pass through the thalamus. One theory is that our senses of taste and smell are the most basic and thus, processed in the most primitive parts of the nervous system, formed before the thalamus.

About 2% of the population under 65 has olfactory problems, while about half of those between 65 and 80 years of age do. This prevalence of olfactory problems increases to about 75% or more in the over-80 population. Many cases of impaired olfaction can be traced to respiratory infections, sinusitis and head trauma.

There is some suggestion that olfactory problems precede cognitive ones. Difficulty detecting and identifying smells occur early in the course of Alzheimer's and other neurodegenerative diseases. Indeed, 70% to 90% of people with Parkinson's disease have some olfactory impairment.

Sometimes, people confuse smell with taste. One way of distinguishing the two is to hold your nose when tasting something, so the smell is significantly reduced or eliminated completely. Because smell is intimately linked to taste, olfactory problems can have a serious impact on nutrition, resulting in the potential failure to detect rotting food or loss of appetite and the enjoyment of eating.

Reduced olfaction is also a risk for other injuries as smell is important in detecting dangers such as fire and toxic chemicals. Given the importance of this sensory system what can be done to enhance it?

Aromatherapy may be an underutilized tool.

The practice of using smells to enhance health has a long history. Aromatherapy has endured partly because it is relatively easy to use, has no side effects and most people are able to tolerate it. In one study, aromatherapy seemed to show benefits even in those people who had lost their psychological perception of smell, an important finding because so many seniors are anosmic (i.e., have lost their sense of smell).

Several different aromas and delivery systems are commonly used to enhance various aspects of wellbeing. The three most popular ways of distributing aromas are through oil burners or diffusers, application to pillows or other materials, and massage. Some people also use a fan to spread the aroma from a burner.

Many aromas are used because they elicit a sense of relaxation and calm. Lavender and lemon oils are particularly noted for their abilities to instill a sense of peace. Some suggest that these aromas also enhance cognitive skills. It is likely that the reduction of any agitation and/or an increase in relaxation would improve mental clarity and performance. Other studies have suggested that aromatherapy can improve sleep, which is a major problem with neurodegenerative disorders. Improved sleep is likely to increase energy, which as we mentioned above has many health benefits.

In one study, the use of lemon balm oil seemed to be associated with behavioral improvements and greater social participation. There is also the suggestion that aromatherapy could be an aid for those at risk for developing pneumonia.

Smell is highly evocative and can be used to stimulate specific memories, emotions or even other physical reactions. Particular aromas, especially novel ones, could be paired with activities to enhance learning and memory. In one classic case study, a child diagnosed with an autoimmune disorder couldn't tolerate the high doses of steroids that are a mainstay of the condition. After the medication was paired repeatedly with a novel aroma, in this case lavender, the aroma itself came to elicit a drug response.

Because smells are easily associated with memories, aromatherapy may be beneficial in the context of cognitive decline.

Ways of Stimulating Olfaction

- Flowers and plants
- Foods and the smells associated with cooking certain foods
- Oils, candles and soaps

Tactile Stimulation

Touch gives us essential information about objects we handle. It also gives us vital information about how others are feeling and can significantly impact mood.

In a series of studies, researchers found that human touch could reliably communicate the positive emotions of joy, love, gratitude and sympathy. Research using the fMRI to monitor different aspects of brain activity suggests that the interpretation of touch is very context-dependent. In other words, how touch is interpreted has a lot to do with circumstances like who is doing the touching, the nature of the relationship, etc.

One value of touch as a form of communication is that it's instant and doesn't require optimal functioning of other senses. Thus, it remains a means of connecting with loved ones who may no longer be able to produce and/or understand language as a result of cognitive decline.

General population studies have found that touching increases cooperation and the positive evaluation of people in such different environments as restaurants, libraries and retail stores. Another study showed that hand-to-hand contact alone was associated with improved quality of life in older adults.

In the context of cognitive decline, one study found that purposeful touching reduced agitation amongst those with dementia in a nursing facility. In another study, participants with Alzheimer's disease felt less depressed and anxious following tactile sensory stimulation. There were also signs that, temporarily at least, they were more socially active and had more energy.

Physical touch as treatment in the form of massage

Massage has been associated with decreased agitation and anxiety. It has also been shown to increase activity in the areas of the brain associated with opioid pain reducers. In one study, six weeks of tactile massage reduced the aggression of participants as well as levels of a physiological marker of stress, chromogranin A (CgA).

Touchy Subject

Touch has become a sensitive issue in contemporary society. Some professional regulations require signed consent before any physical contact can occur. Typically, "safe zones" include the shoulder to the wrist but even then a touch can be misinterpreted. Thus, it is important to communicate prior to massage therapy to ensure that an individual is comfortable with this level of tactile stimulation.

With many types of touch, including massage, there is evidence that the person initiating the touch gets as much benefit as the person receiving it. This is where pet ownership or exposure to animal-assisted therapy is likely to be beneficial; it provides the person with an opportunity to initiate warm touch. Involvement in animal-assisted therapy has been linked to improved socialization and motivation. In addition, tactile stimulation with soft toys or materials can be used to elicit calm.

Some Examples of Tactile Stimulation

- Where appropriate, use touch to convey positive feelings and support
- Encourage seniors to initiate appropriate touch with others and, if applicable, pets
- Consider massage, manicures and pedicures as tactile stimulations that can soothe
- Provide soft "toys" or materials (e.g., blankets) that are comforting to touch

---

From the above it is clear that stimulation of any of the five senses has the potential to relax, and to improve mood, energy and sleep. Thus, sensory stimulation can be used to enhance cooperation and to reduce agitation.

Multi-Sensory Stimulation

Attempts have been made to design systems that stimulate more than one sensory sensation at a time. These multi-sensory approaches stress the value of customizing experiences according to individual needs. To that end, caregivers are encouraged to assess each person's sensory needs and preferences.

As previously discussed, stimulation can include anything from listening to music, to watching different light frequencies, to touching fabrics or soft toys, to getting or giving a massage, to eating or smelling food. An example of a multi-sensory experience could be a massage, given that it engages touch, sound (often spa music plays) and smell (aroma of the oils used). Sometimes, specific rooms are designed to maximize multi-sensory experiences and create a safe, relaxing, environment that can be the setting for various individual and social activities.

While some limited research suggests that mood, behavior, cognition and overall function can all benefit from these approaches, it is unclear how lasting these benefits are. There have been reported reductions in the incidences of psychotic behavior, agitation, disruption and apathy. Multi-sensory approaches thus seem to foster a sense of calm, are generally well-received and can increase communication between clients and their caregivers.

Sensory stimulation can be used to enhance the quality of life of older adults and those with dementia by facilitating memory, instilling a sense of peace, increasing energy, and encouraging social interaction and cooperation.

CHAPTER 5
THE IMPACT OF NUTRITION ON BRAIN HEALTH

Your stomach, intestines, liver and pancreas (hereafter referred to as "the guts") form an incredible system of interconnected chemical factories that reduce foods to microscopic parts to fuel the body. This system almost rivals the brain in its complexity and is often called "the second brain," with good reason. There are millions of cells that connect via pathways directly to the brain; some of these are the pathways by which the brain controls appetite and some are pathways that impact different aspects of brain function. Food, therefore, has an impact on the brain and in this chapter we will look at the role that food plays in overall brain health, with a specific focus on cognitive decline.

First, however, a word of caution is warranted. Claims about the role of food in health have been around for centuries. Many of those claims have not been based on any science and have no empirical support. Unfortunately, that trend continues today. As the population lives longer and concerns about cognitive decline become more prevalent, there will no doubt continue to be spurious claims about "miracle" foods that can enhance cognitive function and slow or even reverse symptoms of dementia. It is important to be able to evaluate those claims to distinguish between those which are valid and those which are baseless. In this chapter we will present a few basic facts that will help you to better contextualize and more critically evaluate the oft-asked question, "What foods are good for brain health?"

What are the effects of a poor diet?

Maintaining a healthy weight is an important factor in overall wellbeing. Worldwide, about 1.4 billion people are overweight, 500 million of which are obese. In addition to lack of exercise, consuming calories in excess, especially in the form of foods high in fat and sugar, can cause obesity. Obesity is a major risk factor for cardiovascular diseases (e.g., heart disease, stroke), diabetes, and other conditions that result in serious disability and sometimes death. A high body-mass index is also associated with cognitive decline and midlife obesity is similarly related to an increased risk of Alzheimer's and vascular dementia.

Metabolic syndrome is diagnosed as a co-occurrence of three out of five of the following medical conditions: abdominal (central) obesity, elevated blood pressure, elevated fasting plasma glucose, high serum triglycerides, and low high-density cholesterol (HDL) levels. In one study, individuals with metabolic syndrome were shown to have an increased risk for developing vascular dementia, while those with diabetes and elevated triglycerides had an increased risk of developing both Alzheimer's and vascular dementia.

Back to the guts...

Your guts do an amazing job crushing, dismantling and demolishing anything that comes their way. The guts are indiscriminating when it comes to the reputation of a food. They don't care whether the food comes from the Mediterranean, the Amazon, Outer Mongolia, or your local market. They don't care whether the food is eaten by Eskimos, Europeans, or cavepersons. They don't care whether the food has its own infomercial, multi-level marketing network or is endorsed by famous doctors. Every food is broken down to molecules;

what is useful is transformed and transported to where it is needed. What isn't useful gets discarded.

When a food is deemed to have beneficial properties there is a tendency to classify that food as "good" and other foods as "bad." This is a problematic way to categorize food, as "good" foods tend to be overvalued. If something is good for you it does not follow that more of it is better. For example, as you will read, the current recommendation is to have at least two servings of fish a week because of its beneficial Omega-3 fatty acid content. You don't have to eat fish at every meal. In fact, doing so might expose you to mercury poisoning and lead you to miss out on nutrients from other sources of lean protein. Similarly, though an exotic berry may pack 20 times more antioxidants than the standard variety, the excess is flushed away by your guts, making your kidneys work harder.

The fact is that most claims about foods are oversimplified or just plain wrong and take advantage of the fact that the average person is neither a gastroenterologist nor a scientist. And even scientists have a tough time getting to the bottom of the real contributions of foods to health.

Most of the quoted research on food's impact on health involves studies in which many people are asked about their food intake retrospectively. There are several problems with this methodology. Most people couldn't reliably tell you what they had to eat yesterday let alone over the past month or longer. In addition, estimation of portions is notoriously unreliable. Moreover, what you drink along with a meal can impact how it is metabolized.

So, what foods are associated with brain health?

There is some suggestion that the Mediterranean diet reduces the risk of developing mild cognitive impairment and Alzheimer's disease. Given the diet's apparent positive effects on cardiovascular health it is reasonable to assume that if the validity of these results were upheld, the diet would also impact the risk for vascular dementia. Let's look at the diet to determine what aspects of it might contribute to decreased risk of cognitive decline.

In the early 1960s, Ancel Keys was a well-publicized proponent of the idea that eating fats resulted in increased serum cholesterol, which in turn led to heart disease. Keys' survey of the diets of seven Western countries led him to conclude that those with the highest fat diets also had the highest incidence of heart disease. Dr. Keys conveniently ignored the contradiction to this hypothesis posed by data from France – France had the highest per-capita consumption of dietary fat but also one of the lowest incidences of heart disease.

Keys' evangelism about the dangers of dietary fats significantly affected recommendations about fats and still impacts perceptions and practices to this day. Later, Keys observed that the high consumption of fat in olive oil was associated with a low incidence of heart disease. He thus concluded that not all fats were the same, and olive oil must fall into what he described as a "good fat" category. Since Keys' observations, we've distinguished "good fats" as unsaturated (e.g., nuts, vegetable oils and fish) and "bad fats" as saturated (e.g., butter, whole-fat milk and cream, ice cream).

Based on the traditional eating habits of the southern Mediterranean cultures, the Mediterranean diet encourages the consumption of fish, fruits, vegetables, whole grains, nuts, and legumes, while limiting the intake of red meat and saturated fats. Rather than seasoning with salt and butter, herbs are used for flavoring.

The real skinny on fats

There's now evidence that the distinction between "good" unsaturated (polyunsaturated and monounsaturated) and "bad" saturated fats may be flawed. In some studies saturated fat has been shown to be more beneficial than polyunsaturated fat. In addition, there's little compelling evidence to suggest that moderate amounts of dietary fat increase the risk of heart disease. Huge amounts of anything, including dietary fat, will lead to weight gain, an increase in fat cells and an increased demand for insulin and other chemicals that can have a very serious effect on the heart and the vascular system.

It is understandable that people would assume that the fat they see on their bodies comes from the fat they see in their foods but this is based on a total misunderstanding of how the body metabolizes and stores food. Any food can become body fat. The fat around your waist could have come from bread or beans, not just from cheese or steak.

The confusion over fats and cholesterol has led to many a person being prescribed a low-fat diet only to discover that overall cholesterol doesn't change. One of these was former president Lyndon Baines Johnson who, after a heart attack was put on a very low-fat, restricted diet. When he couldn't stand it any longer he went back to eating steak and the doctors were confused when his cholesterol went down instead of up.

The key here is excess. You can get fat on a vegetarian diet – although you do have to work a little harder at it. Excess weight is a sign that you are eating too much of at least some things, if not everything. Fats do have more calories than proteins and carbohydrates but that doesn't mean obesity is a result of eating too much fat.

Despite the debate over unsaturated and saturated fats, researchers and doctors agree that trans fats are to be avoided. Trans fats became popular about fifty years ago when doctors started to encourage people to eat them instead of saturated fats (e.g., stick margarine rather than butter). Research now shows that trans fats are very unhealthy and are linked to heart disease. Trans fats stay in the bloodstream longer, raise levels of "bad" (LDL) cholesterol and are incorporated into cell membranes, especially in the arteries, rendering them more susceptible to injury and inflammation.

Trans fats can still be found in cookies, crackers, muffins, French fries, vegetable shortening, chicken nuggets, hard taco shells, frozen dinners and snack foods. The trans-fatty acids from partially hydrogenated vegetable oil should be eliminated from the diet.

Monounsaturated fats
Olive oil	Almonds
Avocado	Peanuts

Polyunsaturated fats
Fatty Fish	Walnuts
Corn Oil	Sunflower seeds
Grape Seed Oil	

Saturated fats
Beef	Ice cream
Lamb	Milk
Pork	Lard

Trans fats
Stick Margarine	Popcorn
Bakery products	Chips
Crackers	Shortening

So what does this all mean for the value of Mediterranean diet?

One of the values of the Mediterranean diet is its emphasis on moderation. The Mediterranean diet advocates eating foods that keep us satiated longer and thus encourages slowly savoring one's meal rather than constantly snacking or overeating.

The Mediterranean diet also emphasizes the consumption of fish and berries, both of which are valuable sources of antioxidants, which are critical for brain health as we'll learn about further into this chapter.

Another value of the Mediterranean diet is its emphasis on fresh foods rather than processed ones. Processed foods typically encourage the storage of fat and thus obesity. And one of the biggest categories of processed foods associated with obesity isn't fat, but certain forms of sugar.

Avoiding artificial sweeteners

Let's take simple table sugar as an example. Table sugar consists of glucose and fructose bonded together. Glucose is the body's fuel, literally used by every cell in the brain and elsewhere in the body. Glucose is so critical that the body has a very elaborate system to absorb, use and store it. If you have too much glucose in your blood, your body stores it in the liver and the muscles as glycogen. If there's not enough glucose, the signal goes out to break down glycogen. When the body tastes sweetness, which it does both on the tongue and in the duodenum (there are taste receptors in your gut), insulin is produced to metabolize the sugar and extract the glucose.

Because insulin is stimulated by the sweet taste of the food, when you eat or drink something with artificial sweetener, the taste buds in your mouth and duodenum signal insulin production. The insulin goes about its job of converting glucose into glycogen to be stored, but as there is no additional glucose actually coming into the system, blood-glucose levels drop. Low blood-glucose levels signal further eating. So the sweetener has encouraged two things: fat storage and further eating.

Fructose is the other component of table sugar. There are two types of fructose and it's important to know the difference because they have different effects on the body. One, natural fructose, is found in fruits and vegetables bound to fiber. As a result, a lot of it is not bioavailable and is simply passed through the gut along with the fiber. The other type of fructose, processed fructose, found in high fructose corn syrup (HFCS) and prevalent in breads, sodas, cookies and processed foods, is not bound to fiber and most of it is rapidly absorbed. Oddly, when you eat a food with HFCS in it, the sweet taste doesn't turn on the insulin factory – it actually turns it off. As insulin is a factor in appetite control, more fructose leads to more eating.

There is variation in how people metabolize free fructose but studies have shown that high fructose intake is associated with increases in fat deposited in the liver and "bad" (LDL) cholesterol as well as insulin resistance. Free fructose has also been shown to have an adverse effect on brain repair in rats. Fructose is a great example of how the same substance can have totally different effects depending on whether it is processed or natural, and whether it is bound to other chemicals or not.

Let's look at those antioxidants we mentioned were good for you.

Free radicals are molecules that are missing some electrons. As a result they try to take electrons off other atoms with which they come in contact. This often sets off a chain reaction with electrons jumping from one molecule to another. When cells, including brain cells, lose electrons they are at risk of becoming dysfunctional and even dying. Some data suggest that damage from free radicals promotes the development of neurodegenerative diseases like Alzheimer's and vascular dementia. Based on this process of decay, Denham Harman proposed the free radical theory of aging in the 1950s. The havoc that free radicals cause is called "oxidative stress." Think of oxidative stress as rust on your brain cells. Clearly rusty neurons are a bad thing.

Antioxidants give free radicals the extra electrons they seek, thus effectively neutralizing them and preventing any further chain reactions. As a result, foods that are rich in antioxidants are generally promoted as good for brain health. Research suggests that long-term intake of antioxidants is associated with slower rates of cognitive decline in seniors. It is also linked to improvements in functioning in those with neurodegenerative diseases. For example, Alzheimer's is associated with increased beta amyloid production, which results in the increased vulnerability of brain cells to damage from free radicals. In one study with rats, an antioxidant (in this case pomegranate juice) improved cognitive functioning and reduced amyloid deposition in the areas of the brain associated with Alzheimer's.

Foods that are packed with antioxidants include blueberries, raspberries, strawberries, blackberries, cranberries, acai berries and elderberries. Other fruits and vegetables that fall into this category include cherries, pomegranates, red grapes, oranges, grapefruits, apples, carrots, broccoli, beets, spinach, kale, cabbage, artichokes, greens and tomatoes. Green and black teas are also antioxidants.

What about Omega-3 fatty acids?

While there is some evidence that Omega-3 fatty acids might help in the management of dementia, this has yet to be proven conclusively. The body uses Omega-3s for building brain cells and controlling blood clotting. Omega-3 fatty acids also slow the buildup of plaque in the arteries and lower blood pressure and triglyceride levels. Since your body cannot make its own Omega-3 fatty acids, you have to get them from your diet.

> Three ounces of salmon contain one to two grams of Omega-3 fatty acids. The typical serving of salmon is six to eight ounces.

Omega-3s consist of EPA (Eicosapentaenoic acid) and DHA (Docosahexaenoic acid). DHA is the most abundant Omega-3 fatty acid in the brain and plays a critical role in both cognitive and emotional functioning, and may slow the progression of both Alzheimer's and vascular dementia by limiting inflammation. There is also the suggestion that DHA increases brain-derived neurotrophic factor (BDNF), which supports existing neurons and encourages the growth of new ones.

The American Heart Association recommends that those with heart disease have one gram of EPA+DHA per day—preferably from fatty fish. Up to four grams daily is recommended for those who need to lower their triglycerides. The Association also recommends eating fish (such as salmon) at least twice a week, even for those with no signs of cardiovascular disease.

Good dietary sources of Omega-3 essential fatty acids include flaxseed oil, walnuts, and fish, in particular wild-caught tuna and salmon, although herring, mackerel, anchovies, and sardines are good sources, as well; just four walnuts a day will significantly increase the Omega-3s in your bloodstream.

Several studies have shown that Omega-3 supplementation (i.e., fish oil capsules) did not lower risk of cardiac death, heart attack or strokes. Thus far, the only known advantage of supplements is for pregnant women.

Just as with many of these recommendations we don't just need to consider ourselves but also the supply chain. For example, in most cases, feeding chickens a diet rich in Omega-3 fatty acids leads them to produce eggs that have higher levels of that beneficial nutrient.

Let's take a look at proteins.

Proteins consist of amino acids that are linked together. Our guts break those links, reducing proteins from hundreds of amino acids down to only two to four amino acids strung together.

> Our body makes 85% of the protein its needs. The other 15% comes from food we consume.

The body can make most of the amino acids it needs to build proteins or repair tissues, but some must be obtained directly from our diet. These are called essential amino acids and include: isoleucine, leucine, methionine, phenylalanine, threonine, tryptophan, valine, histidine and tyrosine.

All meats, poultry and fish are considered complete proteins because they contain all of the essential amino acids that we need. Vegetarians have to work harder and mix foods to get complete proteins because no plant contains all the essential amino acids.

Now, some of these protein food sources have extra benefits. For example, fish, being high in Omega-3s have anti-inflammatory properties as described above, and that may be why some research suggests that they reduce the risk of dementia and are a better protein source. However, that doesn't mean that other protein sources, such as red meat, are necessarily "bad." In other words, the current thinking that eating fish twice a week is sufficient for health benefits doesn't preclude one from eating meat and other protein sources. Nuts are another great source of protein, especially because they offer antioxidant properties that other sources of protein do not.

Are "carbs" bad?

Carbohydrates have several functions, not the least of which is to provide energy (in the form of glucose) for the brain and body. Chemically, carbohydrates are chains of sugars and can fall into two categories. Simple carbohydrates like the table sugar referenced earlier provide calories but few nutrients while complex carbohydrates like whole-grain breads provide fiber, vitamins and minerals.

Simple carbohydrates are broken down and absorbed more quickly than complex ones. As a result blood-glucose levels can rise rapidly. As insulin deals with this rise, the result is a fall in blood-glucose, which can stimulate more eating. This can feel like an "addiction," as people cycle between high and low blood-glucose levels. When fructose is added to this picture it, too, can stimulate appetite as mentioned earlier. Some researchers believe that this cycle contributes to diabetes.

With complex carbohydrates, sugar is extracted more slowly, resulting in much less pronounced rises (and falls) in blood-glucose with, therefore, less stimulation of appetite. The fiber in these carbohydrates also serves to fill the stomach and promote stomach stretch; fiber can be thought of as a key that turns off appetite.

In general, the complex carbohydrates are favored for overall health, including brain health. This, of course, doesn't mean that you can't eat simple carbohydrates but that when you do, you should combine them with slower digesting foods (there are those fruits and vegetables again) or foods that moderate the sweetness in the carbs.

Vitamins and minerals are important, but why?

Vitamins and minerals are essential to helping the body fight free radicals and for optimal cell function.

Most vitamins and minerals necessary for healthy functioning can be found in everyday foods and only small amounts are required. Indeed, in larger amounts they can be toxic. For example, some minerals, such as iron, are called "heavy metals" and over-exposure can result in toxicity. It has also been established that aluminum exposure can lead to Alzheimer's-like neurological problems.

B Vitamins comprise 8 of the 13 essential vitamins and, although chemically distinct from one another, often exist in the same foods. Certain B vitamins have been shown to be potentially effective in lowering elevated plasma homocysteine concentrations, which is possibly associated with cognitive impairment. One recent study suggested that B vitamin supplementation can slow the decline of specific regions in the medial temporal lobe that can be characteristic of Alzheimer's.

The role of Vitamin B1 (thiamin) is to facilitate the conversion of carbohydrates into energy. Thiamin deficiencies show up in alcoholics and manifest as confusion, fatigue and even psychosis. Extreme forms appear as Korsakoff's syndrome and Wernicke's encephalopathy, both of which result in severe memory disturbances. These conditions typically can be reversed with vitamin B1 supplementation.

Vitamin D deficiency has also been shown to be related to cognitive impairment caused by free radicals and the value of its neuro-protective effect in the context of several conditions like Alzheimer's, Parkinson's and MS has been noted.

A diet high in natural vitamin C and vitamin E is recommended as both act as antioxidants, fighting free radicals and supporting cognitive health.

Some key vitamins and minerals

Vitamin/Mineral	Benefits	Some Sources
Vitamin A (can be converted from beta carotene)	Supports vision, skin and tissue health	Beef, liver, eggs, fish, sweet potatoes, carrots
Vitamin B1 (Thiamin)	Supports skin, hair, muscles and brain health	Pork chops, ham, soy milk
Vitamin B2 (Riboflavin)	Supports skin, hair, blood and brain health	Milk, yogurt, cheese
Vitamin B3 (Niacin)	Supports skin, blood cells, brain and nervous system health	Meat, poultry, fish, whole grains, mushrooms
Vitamin B12 (Cobalamin)	Assists in making new cells, and breaking down some fatty acids and amino acids; protects nerve cells; helps make red blood cells	Meat, poultry, fish, milk, cheese, eggs
Vitamin C (Ascorbic acid)	Helps make collagen, serotonin and norepinephrine; acts as an antioxidant; strengthens the immune system	Citrus fruits, potatoes, broccoli, spinach, tomatoes
Vitamin D (Calciferol)	Helps maintain levels of calcium and phosphorous to strengthen bones	Fortified milk and cereals, fatty fish
Vitamin E (Alpha-tocopherol)	Acts as an antioxidant	Nuts, wheat germ, leafy green vegetables, whole grains, vegetable oils
Vitamin K (Phylloquinone, menadione)	Activates proteins and calcium essential to blood clotting	Cabbage, kale, liver, eggs, spinach, broccoli, sprouts
Copper	Helps make red blood cells; involved in iron metabolism	Liver, shellfish, nuts, whole grains, beans
Manganese	Helps form bones; helps metabolize amino acids, cholesterol and carbohydrates	Nuts, legumes, whole grains
Selenium	Acts as an antioxidant; helps regulate thyroid hormones	Seafood, walnuts

This is not an exhaustive list. For more complete information please visit **www.health.harvard.edu/newsweek/Listing_of_vitamins.htm**.

A note on supplements

Outside of malnourishment and pregnancy, the use of supplements to enhance health or protect against chronic disease remains controversial. For example, gingko biloba has been touted as a supplement that can enhance memory and concentration but there's little scientific evidence that it produces any clinically meaningful effects. Research data have been inconsistent and the long-term effects of supplementation are unknown. Dietary supplements are not regulated by the Food and Drug Administration, and therefore claims made by manufacturers are unregulated.

Now that we've discussed food, let's move on to how what we drink can impact our brains.

There is no question that heavy alcohol consumption is harmful and has the potential to be seriously toxic to the brain. The specific condition of Korsakoff's psychosis that can be seen in heavy alcohol users is marked by the loss of neurons and deficits in declarative memory.

Alcohol impacts the hippocampus and other areas of the brain that are implicated in memory and learning. That's why blackouts and memory problems can occur when you have had too much to drink. Given the potential damage, one would expect that the recommended alcohol consumption for seniors, and especially for those already experiencing cognitive decline, would be set at an extremely low level, if recommended at all. However, studies in the last few years have suggested that moderate alcohol consumption might be beneficial for reducing the risk of heart disease and possibly enhancing brain function. These studies need closer examination.

Most compare non-drinkers, light or moderate drinkers, and heavy drinkers on a variety of health outcomes. Typically, light/moderate drinkers fare better than non-drinkers. Leaving aside the issue of the reliability of individual's report of his or her consumption, there are other major problems with this research. The "abstainers" may not be a fair comparison against which to measure the impacts of drinking, as there can be many health reasons for their abstinence. They may be recovering alcoholics or drug addicts, people on medications like sedatives that are not to be mixed with alcohol or people trying to lose weight – people who may not be in ideal health.

Some studies have moved beyond consumption to specific types of alcohol. Resveratrol, an ingredient in red wine, has been touted as a brain-boosting chemical. This has been shown in the laboratory. However, there is a huge difference between a demonstration in a laboratory and the real world of the human gut. Dr. Terry Simpson, a leading gastro-intestinal specialist and surgeon with years of experience understanding digestion and the metabolism of food, suggests in his book *Gutted! The Great Food Hoax: What food can and can't do for your health* that to get any heart or brain protective benefits from resveratrol one would have to drink 2000 bottles of red wine a day! Cheers!

No responsible health agency has encouraged people to start drinking alcohol in order to boost health. Very light alcohol consumption probably doesn't do any harm, but it's questionable whether it does you any good.

- Alcohol stimulates appetite, so you can eat more than you planned

- Willpower dissolves in alcohol, so that you can eat more than you planned

- As we age, we tend to lose body weight, reducing tolerance to our habitual levels of alcohol consumption

- Alcohol consumption is actually discouraged or even contraindicated when taking many types of medications

- Alcohol consumption could lead to balance issues and falls, a leading cause of injury for seniors

The impact of a particular amount of alcohol is dependent on a variety of factors like weight, so it is difficult to give precise amount recommendations. Drinking every day is not a good idea for anyone. A very rough guideline for the maximum limits for seniors would be no more than three times a week and no more than the equivalent of 8 ounces of wine (two small glasses) in any one day. Anyone using alcohol, even recreationally, should disclose this to his or her physician to ensure optimal health.

Does that morning cup'o joe give your brain energy for the day?

Research has suggested that caffeine might be beneficial for brain health. One study suggested that consumption of three to five cups of coffee per day in the middle-aged was associated with a 65% lower rate of developing Alzheimer's or other forms of dementia in later life. Daily consumption of coffee also may reduce the risk for developing Parkinson's disease and diabetes. However, caffeine can cause irritability and insomnia, so caution is urged. Moreover, it is best if caffeine comes from coffee or tea and not sodas, which carry other dietary risks such as high levels of free fructose. Contrary to what was once thought, caffeine is NOT a diuretic, so concerns about dehydration no longer apply. Which raises the subject of hydration...

Water is critical for effective body and brain function. Dehydration can cause confusion and mental fogginess. It is best to consume water slowly throughout the day, as glugging several ounces at a time is likely to stimulate the excretion of the water. Carrying a bottle of water with you can be inconvenient but is the best way of getting constant hydration. The typical recommendation is 64 fluid ounces a day though that can vary depending on numerous variables, like ambient temperature, levels of activity, etc.

That was a lot of information. What are the main takeaways?

There is a sufficient scientific base to support the argument that some foods or diets can boost brain health, though the touting of specific foods as "miracle foods" should arouse suspicion. In addition to adopting a healthy diet, maintaining a healthy weight can help in delaying or offsetting vascular conditions and other mechanisms that impact brain function.

Despite the fads and pseudoscience that abound in the nutrition "pop-science" it is fair to say that at this time, the scientific evidence does support the following:

- Trans fats are bad and should be avoided

- Free fructose is likely to have a negative impact on cardiovascular and brain health

- Alcohol consumption should be avoided for those who show signs of cognitive decline

- Brain superfoods like fish, nuts, dark chocolate, blueberries and olive oil help reduce the risk of heart disease and diabetes, and promote blood flow to the brain

- Moderation is critical. You can have too much of a good thing – and a bad thing

- Drink plenty of water each day

- Saturated fats like red meat and ice-cream are not inherently bad and can be eaten in moderation

- Taking supplements is not the same as getting nutrients from food

- It's better to have your food processed in your gut than processed in the factory

CHAPTER 6
EXERCISE AND DEMENTIA

Note: Before beginning any exercise program it is a good idea to talk with your doctor about any limitations you may have. Once you begin an exercise routine, maintain regular visits with your doctor in order to ensure your continued health and wellness. For those with multiple co-morbidities, the American College of Sports Medicine (2010) specifically recommends evaluation by a physician prior to the initiation of an exercise program to learn about specific safety tips and guidelines for exercises.

In this chapter we will consider the role of exercise in preserving brain function.

Most people know that exercise is beneficial for overall health, which is why Nancy, Franny and Jane (our friends from *Chapter 3*) were walking around the lake one morning.

"So how long have you guys been doing this?" asked Jane.

"I've been an exerciser most of my life," said Franny. "I can't imagine not being active. I think I would go out of my mind if I didn't move. I know that when I can't exercise, it drives me nuts. It's a lifesaver."

"Honestly, I started when my dad was diagnosed with Alzheimer's," said Nancy. "Somebody told me that exercise could lower my risk of getting the disease and that was motivation enough for me."

Humans were made to move. In fact, our ancestors survived in part because they could outrun and outwalk most other mammals over long distances; there may have been faster species but humans possess a high level of endurance. In this way, natural selection drove early humans to become more athletic, developing shorter toes, inner-ear mechanisms to maintain balance and other unique anatomical structures, such as the Achilles heal, which allow for running long distances and continued physical activity. So, exercise and movement have been key to survival. But, is Franny accurate when she says it is a "life-saver?" And is Nancy misinformed by thinking exercise can prevent her from getting Alzheimer's?

The perils of moving toward less movement

First, let us make the distinction between activity and exercise. Physical activity means movement of the skeletal muscles. This can include walking from one room to another, stretching to pick something up or carrying a food tray from a buffet bar back to your table. Exercise also involves movement but it is planned movement designed to challenge the body in some way. So swimming, lifting a weight, balancing on one leg or walking a mile are all considered forms of exercise.

As we age we may be faced with physical limitations, which reduce our ability to exercise. For example, loss of muscle mass and bone density are normal consequences of the aging process. Low energy and other psychological conditions like depression, can also limit motivation. In addition, many seniors and/or their caregivers may not be aware of which forms of physical activity are appropriate. There can also be practical limitations, such as the ability to get to a gym or an exercise facility safely.

Barriers to Exercise

- Limited access to facilities
- Lower Energy
- Depression
- Physical disability
- Concerns about safety

There is no question that technological developments have contributed to individuals becoming more sedentary. This increasingly sedentary lifestyle is considered a global health challenge associated with many adverse outcomes.

Lack of exercise is implicated in 16% of all deaths for men and women. Inactivity is a major factor in the development of obesity and the associated conditions of type-2 diabetes and cardiovascular disease. Exercise also seems to have a bearing on the risk for neurodegenerative diseases, as Nancy mentioned. Those who do not exercise in midlife have about a 250% greater risk of developing Alzheimer's disease than those who do exercise. Less fit people also have less grey matter in various areas of the brain including the frontal and temporal regions, which affect executive function, language skills and other cognitive processes. Thus, exercise can have beneficial effects in a number of domains including cognition, function, physical health and mental health.

The impact of exercise on physical fitness

Falls are the leading cause of both fatal and nonfatal injuries among older adults. In addition to physical risk factors including mobility and balance issues, cognitive risk factors, particularly impaired executive functioning, are associated with falls. The good news is that research shows that exercise not only improves physical functioning but also executive functioning.

Diminished balance is a major problem for the senior population as falls are an ever-present risk. Those with dementia have a risk of falling that is eight times greater than those without it. Regular exercise increases muscle and bone mass, and improves balance. One study suggested that balance exercises reduced falls by 42% amongst one group of senior participants. Maintaining strong bones and flexible muscles will also help you maintain your independence for a longer period of time.

There are specific exercises that are designed to improve balance and mobility, and thereby confidence in independent movement. For example, combining aerobic activity with upper and lower body conditioning twice a week for an hour improved stamina and agility as well as mood in one study. Physical status in general was improved in a group of 153 people with Alzheimer's, who also showed benefits in mood and function, effects that lasted at least two years.

One study of people with Alzheimer's showed that a four month community-based program of daily walking, balance and strength training improved both cognition and functioning. The same result was found in a study of 150 people at high risk for cognitive decline. The exercise regimen that was used in the study was a once-a-week 90-minute session that included 30 minutes of walking and 60 minutes of group-based exercises.

One research team found that balance and strength training improved executive functioning among seniors with a recent history of falls. The group identified three benefits in cognitive functioning:

- Reduction of serum homocysteine, which is associated with impaired cognitive performance, Alzheimer's and cerebral white matter lesions

- Increased concentrations of insulin-like growth factor 1, which improves cognitive performance, and promotes neuronal growth, survival and differentiation

- Moderation of the development of sarcopenia, which is the loss of muscle and onset of frailty that is associated with increased falls and fracture risk as well as physical disability

Some cite a fear of falling as a reason for not engaging in exercise; it is important for seniors with these concerns to speak with a physician, physical therapist or experienced trainer in order to develop a plan that suits their needs and any physical limitations.

More on the impact of exercise on cognitive function

Our brains were shaped and sharpened by movement. There are numerous studies which strongly indicate that regular exercise, even walking, can improve mental abilities across the lifespan.

A twelve-year study involving more than 30,000 people suggested a positive correlation between high levels of exercise and cognitive health and that even low to moderate exercise offered some protection against cognitive decline.

Another study found significantly improved cognitive performance on tests of memory and verbal reasoning following six months of moderate or high intensity resistance training in senior subjects. Resistance training involves the use of weight to challenge and strengthen muscles.

Several studies have focused on exercise regimens that involve both resistance training and endurance training, like walking. In one research study involving healthy senior women, those involved in a program of 30 minutes of endurance training followed by 60 minutes of strength, flexibility and balance training performed as well on cognitive tasks as the cognitive stimulation group that had taken a computer course on the use of software for a variety of typical tasks (e.g., writing, calculating, surfing the Internet, emailing, drawing, image editing). The scores of the control group declined compared to the exercise and cognitive groups.

Aerobic, endurance activity is beneficial in promoting heart and vascular health. Aerobic activity also increases levels of brain-derived neurotrophic factor (BDNF), a protein that pharmaceutical companies have being trying to bottle for the last three decades. BDNF (as mentioned in *Chapter 5*) seems heavily involved in preserving cognitive capacities; it can be conceptualized as "fertilizer for brain cells," promoting tissue health and growth throughout the body.

Other research using mice found that aerobic activity actually decreased beta amyloid plaque levels in the brain and long-term running seemed to improve learning. Similarly, people with Alzheimer's who are in better shape have shown less brain atrophy than their less active counterparts. One suggestion is that the improved cerebral blood flow that occurs with aerobic activity can promote healing in the damaged areas of the brain such as the hippocampus (if you recall, that's the brain structure that manages memory). Aerobic exercise also increases nitric oxide levels, which may also help to break up amyloid plaques.

Because of the major impact on brain health, ideal exercise programs include an aerobic component. For example, in a review of several studies, walking combined with strength training had the best results in improving attention and processing speed as well as working memory.

Aerobic activity might not be possible for many seniors but that should not deter from all activity. One small study with very frail participants suffering from dementia showed positive results with a twice-weekly 45-minute session of strengthening, coordination, balance, flexibility and stamina exercises. Another study looked at a home-based activity program that required participants to do 150 minutes a week of activity, mostly walking. The participants that were working out showed significantly better cognitive scores throughout the trial, with better delayed recall and improved clinical ratings. Perhaps most important, the benefits were maintained at a one-year follow up.

There's some suggestion that women might experience more cognitive benefit from exercise than men. This was the conclusion from one study of people with mild cognitive impairment. Cortisol, a stress hormone that can impact cognition, was found to be reduced more in the women in this study. However, while there might be some gender-specific variations in response to different exercises, this in no way means that exercise is not also extremely beneficial to men.

Some studies have looked at combining both an exercise component and a cognitive one and have found increased value. That raises the question of whether exercise has a generalized long-term benefit and/or a short-term benefit. In other words, does exercise improve learning ability in the immediate period following activity? Would doing aerobic exercise facilitate learning later in the day? No one knows for sure. In any case, exercise is linked with brain health.

The impact of exercise on mood

It has been known for some time that exercise has a beneficial effect on mood, especially in the context of depression. Even as new medications like Prozac were being released onto the market in the mid-1980s, practitioners were touting the benefits of exercise as an antidepressant. Exercise raises the levels of serotonin, a neurotransmitter that modulates mood – the same goal of common SSRI (Selective Serotonin Reuptake Inhibitors) antidepressant medications. Exercise also raises levels of dopamine, the neurotransmitter associated with motivation and pleasure. The hurdle with exercise as a treatment is that depressed people, by the very nature of their condition, often find it difficult to summon the motivation to exercise.

Rates of depression are high among those with cognitive impairment and use of many of the standard antidepressant medications is discouraged because it can increase the risk of bone loss and falls.

Exercise involves some level of social interaction with either the other participants and/or the instructor as well as some cognitive challenge in following along with instructions, not to mention the initiation of movement itself. In addition, exercise is associated with improved appetite and better quality sleep, two behaviors that can increase energy. A regular physical activity might also provide some much needed structure and sense of purpose, which conceivably would boost mood and quality of life. Some research suggests that exercise-related improvements in mood could be long-lasting.

In general, exercise has been found to be a potent way of lifting mood, when you can motivate yourself or others to do it. One way of encouraging participation is to embed movement and exercise in a variety of other activities.

Multi-modal approaches

As we have seen elsewhere in this book, combining cognitive, sensory and social activities provides greater opportunities for challenge than each does alone; adding exercise or physical movement would enhance such activities even more. For example, you might join a neighborhood walking group or start one with your friends the way Jane, Nancy and Franny did.

One value of adding exercise as part of a multi-modal approach is that physical movement becomes part of ongoing activities rather than a separate, and potentially less desirable, "exercise session." Thus, participation is likely to be higher and sustained over a longer period of time. Commitment to an exercise regimen also depends largely on the support and encouragement seniors receive from their caregivers, when applicable.

How can caregivers help?

The caregiver is a critical variable in the quality of life of someone suffering from a neurodegenerative disorder. Whether the caregiver is a professional from a home care agency or a family member, his or her attitudes, moods and behaviors can have a significant effect on the person for whom he or she is caring. If the caregiver is overworked and experiencing burnout, he or she will be less able to provide opportunities for stimulation, whereas an upbeat, energetic caregiver is likely to encourage participation in different types of activities, including exercise. Any exercise-induced functional improvements in clients or loved ones are likely to make life easier for caregivers.

As a caregiver, one way you can engage your client or loved one in activities is to participate in them yourself (e.g., "let's stretch together"). You'll reap the health benefits of exercise, socialization and cognitive stimulation as well! Exercise can help relieve some of the stress associated with caregiving, which can be debilitating not just for the caregiver but also for the person receiving care.

One study actually looked at whether caregiver education on behavior modification and exercise improved clients' abilities and reduced the burden of care. Data at three months suggested improvements in functioning that seemed to be maintained for at least two years.

Nancy was surprised to learn that the assisted living facility where her dad was residing had encouraged him to start lifting weights. When she spoke to the person leading the activity, she heard how important resistance training seemed to be. The next day, Nancy suggested to her friends that they start lifting some weights, too.

"Hey, I have no desire to develop muscles. I'm not a bodybuilder," said Jane.

"This is not about building muscles; it's about preserving them," said Nancy. "Now that we're over sixty we have to work really hard to preserve what we've got. Lifting light weights will increase our aerobic capacity, and improve our fatty acid metabolism and our bone and joint health."

"She's right," said Franny. "I just do not get the same kick out of lifting weights that I do from aerobic activity."

"I've found a fun work-out video that has some upbeat music and if we do it together, it will be more fun. What do you think?" said Nancy.

"We should do it. We're working our leg muscles when we walk but we're doing nothing for our upper body strength. Loading the dishwasher just doesn't count. Let's do it girls," said Franny.

A body in motion

It is clear that exercise can benefit almost everybody at any age. Ideally a comprehensive activity program would include exercises designed to improve strength, flexibility, balance and endurance.

> ## *Tai Chi and Yoga*
>
> Tai chi and yoga are activities that include stretching, balance and strength exercises and can be modified to accommodate different ability levels. The fact that these activities are typically done in group sessions and also encourage relaxation and controlled breathing makes them ideal for overall health.

Recommendations for the frequency of exercise vary, but in general, about 30 minutes of moderately intense aerobic exercise every day, or about the same time of more intense exercise every other day, can reap benefits. Although the incorporation of general physical activity into daily life can be helpful, it is not seen as being as beneficial as specific exercise routines. Taking an exercise class from a trained instructor who can monitor physical activity, correct form and motivate individuals to push a little harder is helpful.

Intensity is also an important consideration. Obviously people will have different comfort and ability levels, but in general, the more intense the level of exercise that can safely be done, the better.

Suggestions for adapting exercise routines for those with some form of cognitive impairment include reducing group size, modifying exercises so they can be done from a seated position, increasing instructor-participant interaction and incorporating activities that participants are familiar with (e.g. the use of a basketball for those who once played the sport). Dementia is not a contraindication to exercise; rather, individuals with dementia stand to make gains across multiple areas of functioning, including cognition.

CHAPTER 7
STRESS, PSYCHOLOGICAL SYMPTOMS AND COGNITIVE IMPAIRMENT

In this chapter we will consider the psychological symptoms that can accompany the diagnosis of dementia and how they can impact the life of the individual and the caregiver. We will also review some of the techniques that are available to manage these conditions.

The bad news: stress is unavoidable...

Stress is an inevitable part of life. Research dating back 50 years to the development of the classic Holmes and Rahe life stress questionnaire showed that any change in life circumstances can be stressful – even positive changes. The most stressful events were ones in which people felt out of control or helpless, such as the death of a loved one.

Increased stress levels and negative mood states can be common in individuals with cognitive impairment, which itself represents a significant life change over which a person has little control. There is also some evidence suggesting that stress itself could hasten the onset of neurodegenerative diseases. One longitudinal study found that increased stress was associated with the risk of developing Alzheimer's disease later in life.

Particular symptoms of stress are also commonly associated with dementia. Collectively, these symptoms are called the Behavioral and Psychological Symptoms of Stress and Disease, or BPSD. These symptoms typically include apathy, depression, agitation/aggression, irritability, delusions, anxiety and impulse control issues. Almost two-thirds of those with dementia score higher in the measurement of symptoms of stress than those without dementia.

The good news...

Being aware of the health risks associated with increased stress levels is often a motivating factor for many to make a conscious effort to allow more time for relaxation and calm. While living with dementia or having a loved one who has some form of cognitive impairment can be incredibly stressful, being aware of the various psychological manifestations of the disease is the first step to improving quality of life.

So what exactly are the common psychiatric and mood conditions associated with dementia?

Depression

Depression is characterized by feelings of worthlessness, hopelessness and guilt. As one might expect, and has been discussed elsewhere in this book, depression is associated with greater cognitive and functional deficits as well as an increased risk of hospitalization, suicide and increased caregiver stress, ultimately resulting in burnout.

The identification and diagnosis of depression can vary depending on the environment in which an individual resides. In epidemiological studies, the prevalence rates of diagnosed depression in those with dementia living in nursing homes range from 9% to 30% even though the prevalence of depressive symptoms is estimated at closer to 65% in that environment.

One study suggested that for more than half of those diagnosed with dementia, depression was a new diagnosis (i.e., they had not been previously diagnosed with the condition), suggesting that the dementia was associated with the depression. More important, those who were depressed were more cognitively impaired, had more behavioral problems and reported pain more often than those who were not diagnosed with depression. In one study, depressed participants with dementia performed significantly worse on measures of perception, attention, memory, calculation and language than their peers with dementia who did not also have depression.

Depression might also be a precursor to dementia. A history of depression is associated with a 150% increase in the risk of developing dementia in those over the age of 65. A depressed twin is three times more likely to develop dementia than his or her non-depressed counterpart.

Apathy

Apathy is often misdiagnosed as depression, and it should be noted that some experts argue that the distinction is too blurred to truly separate the two conditions, especially in older adults where the conditions can co-occur. Typically, however, apathy refers to a general lack of motivation, energy and reduced emotional response that does not meet clinical diagnostic criteria for depression. Research has ranked apathy as the most common symptom of Alzheimer's, with one study suggesting a prevalence of 92% in those with the disease.

Those with a form of cognitive impairment may need more prompting. Caregivers need to understand that the people they are caring for may be apathetic and not oppositional. They will need patience in dealing with troublesome behaviors and will need to use prompts to cue and motivate their care recipients. The goal is to have the person do something, even if he or she can't perform that task very well. For the apathetic person it is about action, not accuracy.

Anxiety

Reports suggest that approximately 5% to 20% of those with dementia have an anxiety disorder, while the presence of anxiety symptoms may be as high as 70%. Anxiety is more common in both vascular dementia and frontotemporal dementia and is less prevalent in the later stages of Alzheimer's. In the sense that anxiety is often anticipatory, it might be reduced by a decreased capacity to project into the future – a characteristic common in those with more advanced forms of cognitive impairment.

Anxiety in individuals with dementia is associated with decreased functional and cognitive abilities. However, anxiety may not always be diagnosed. For one thing, anxiety can be confused with depression. Moreover, some of the symptoms of anxiety like restlessness, poor concentration and fatigue, can be mistaken for symptoms of the dementia.

Sleep Dysfunctions

The loss of energy that can accompany depression, apathy and anxiety can lead to problems with sleeping. Sometimes these issues lead to insomnia, daytime napping and sundowning, a syndrome marked by nocturnal agitation, confusion, and wandering which is common among those with dementia. Naturally, sleepiness can exacerbate cognitive and functional difficulties. In an earlier chapter, light therapy was mentioned as a way of maintaining a healthy sleep-wake cycle. Other strategies include limiting the time spent in bed when not sleeping and reducing daytime napping.

---

7 Tips for Better Sleep

- Establish a regular bed time
- Avoid napping during the day
- Avoid caffeine, nicotine and alcohol 4 -6 hours before bedtime
- Exercise in the afternoon, not before bedtime
- Make the bed and environment comfortable and calming
- Eliminate noise and lighting
- Practice relaxation techniques before bed

Psychosis

Delusions and hallucinations are more common in the later stages of dementia. Hallucinations involve seeing, hearing or smelling something that others do not sense. Delusions are fixed, false beliefs. Some common delusions among those with a form of cognitive impairment include the belief that people are stealing from them, that various people are impostors and fears of abandonment. Depressed people are more prone to delusions, which seem to be highest among those with Alzheimer's than those with other forms of dementia.

Other Symptoms

Although other symptoms like eating dysfunctions and sexual disinhibition are occasionally reported there is less evidence about the prevalence of these problems in the context of dementia specifically. Still, these behaviors can be very distressing to both individuals and their caregivers.

Rather than assume they are unavoidable manifestations of the disease, caregivers should note concerning behaviors and speak with the individual's physician about them to explore pharmacological or behavioral modifications.

What can be done to improve mental wellbeing?

Regardless of the condition, an integrated approach to treatment involving all those who play a key role in the individual's care is the optimal approach. Repetition of the treatment message is not just helpful for consistency but can also help compensate for cognitive difficulties that might lead to the person forgetting the treatment plan and objective. Using this coordinated approach, one study showed that 42% of residents in a care facility successfully reduced their BPSD symptoms.

Treatment approaches need to be individualized to account for each person's strengths and weaknesses. They should also have very specific, realistic and measurable goals such as improvement of working memory, the reduction of agitated outbursts or more night-time sleep.

Medications
As mentioned elsewhere in this book, drug treatments need to be used with caution. Side effects, drug interactions and overdose are all potential dangers for anyone on medication, but especially for seniors and those with an existing cognitive condition.

Nonetheless, medications are often prescribed. As mentioned in *Chapter Two*, some medications can exacerbate cognitive decline and others can lead to drowsiness or can impact memory. Given such concerns, attention is turned to non-pharmacological interventions.

Non-Pharmacological Treatments
Behavioral Therapy is based on the idea that rewarding positive behavior will increase its occurrence. Thus, when someone acts appropriately he or she is given a reward, which could be anything from verbal praise and affirmation to some

material benefit like a trip to a favorite restaurant or museum. Undesirable behavior is not reinforced and might be ignored or actively discouraged.

Use of this technique has been shown to be effective in reducing verbal and physical aggression as well as improving wandering and incontinence in those with cognitive impairment. This treatment works best as a team approach – it is not helpful if one person is ignoring a positive behavior and another is reinforcing it. Consistency is crucial, which may mean special training for caregivers. In one study, such caregiver training led to a reduction of problem behaviors, an improvement that was maintained at a six-month follow-up.

Cognitive Behavioral Therapy (CBT) is a treatment that involves considering the individual's thoughts, perceptions and attitudes, and either validating them or identifying and correcting the flaws in them. CBT could be helpful in the early stages of diagnosis but since it requires a fair degree of insight and a reasonable level of cognitive functioning, it may not be as useful in the later stages of dementia. As the disease progresses, CBT could be used to help caregivers by examining their thoughts about their roles and concerns, and thus helping them adapt to changing circumstances.

Problem Adaptation Therapy is a home or facility-based intervention that involves training caregivers to identify and implement ways of engaging cognitively challenged, depressed individuals. Making environmental changes, using cues and prompts, and breaking tasks down into small steps are just some of the ways caregivers are taught to circumvent the individual's difficulties.

Interpersonal Psychotherapy, like CBT, requires insight and at least moderate cognitive functioning to be effective. It can be valuable in helping seniors with anxiety and depression in the early stages of cognitive decline. Psychotherapy can include giving support, problem-solving, and helping the individual to access and express feelings.

Reminiscence Therapy is another technique that might help temporarily relieve depression and/or anxiety. This form of therapy encourages people to recall positive aspects of their lives. It can be accompanied by music or other sensory cues that can prompt recall of past events. It can be done one-on-one using events in the individual's own life or in groups referencing historical or cultural events of a given era.

Encouraging individuals to record a story of their lives in either pictures or words can also be helpful in stimulating recall as well as creating a sense of purpose. Many caregivers also report finding this type of activity enjoyable and helpful in bonding with the individual.

Pet Therapy can also improve mood. In *Chapter 4*, we mentioned the value of having a pet or being exposed to one from both a tactile and social perspective. In one small study, having a pet in the home was associated with decreased verbal aggression in individuals with dementia. Of course, it is important to ensure that the pet will be safe and well cared for in the home. If having a full-time pet is too big of a responsibility, even having designated "pet cuddling time," where a loved one or neighbor stops by with a pet can be a good way to incorporate pet therapy into an individual's care plan.

Environmental Modifications can also be helpful. As individuals decline they may be less able to cope with environmental stimulation. Limiting stimulation through simple acts, such as removing televisions and other sources of noise, speaking in lower volumes, moderating ambient light levels and decorating in neutral colors, can all reduce sensory load and stress.

Brain Training is gaining popularity as a legitimate way to improve several aspects of brain function and symptoms of BPSD. Neurofeedback, or brain biofeedback, has been around for forty years but is only recently getting more attention because computerization now allows for it to be delivered in an office or even a home environment. Neurofeedback is a way of retraining different areas of the brain and has been shown to be effective for a number of conditions like anxiety, depression, pain, and migraines, to name just a few.

The most popular version of the technique is based on an analysis of brain waves using a variant of the electro-encephalo-gram (EEG). Electrodes attached to the individual's scalp provide information about brain activity like which brain waves are dominant, whether those waves are running high or low compared to a standardized database matched for age and gender, how well the right and left hemispheres are communicating with each other, and so forth. Based on this "brain-map" a protocol is generated that determines which areas of the brain are best targeted for biofeedback.

The actual brain training procedure simply requires participants to sit in a relaxing chair and watch a video and/or listen to music wearing a headset and specially adapted glasses that flash at a certain electronic frequency. As the individual watches the video or listens to the music, information about his or her brainwave frequency in the targeted area is fed into the computer. It has long been established that the brain will match the frequency of flashing light – what is called "photic driving" – so to help the brain reach a desired frequency, for example the relaxed wakefulness of a 9 Hz alpha wave, the glasses will flash at 9 Hz.

Software sets the desired frequency ranges for the targeted brain areas. When the areas are in the desired range, the music or video plays normally; when they are out of the range the video or music fades. This cues the brain to get back to the training range and when it does, it is rewarded with the resumption of normal video and sound function. This retraining system therefore uses operant conditioning as it rewards the brain for being in the desired brainwave state, reinforcing the behavior.

Brain Waves		
The frequency range and associated states of consciousness of the four most common brain waves		
Delta	1-4 cycles per second	Deep sleep
Theta	4-8 cycles per second	Light sleep/deep meditation
Alpha	8-13 cycles per second	Relaxed wakefulness
Beta	13-30 cycles per second	Cognitive processing, stress

This method requires little of people except to sit in a comfortable chair and view a video. The technology can actually be very enjoyable. The videos used are entertaining and interesting and can seem more like a videogame. For example, in one variation, the person can see an aerial view of some famous landmarks such as Stonehenge. The use of flashing light can preclude those with a history of epilepsy but other than that, the technique has few risks and is non-invasive. Sessions last about thirty minutes. The number of sessions required for significant reduction in symptoms is different for each person, but typically ranges from 20 to 40 sessions. The changes are often maintained without further sessions over a period of years.

There are numerous variations on the concept of brain training. Audio-Visual Entrainment (AVE) is a portable device that also uses sound and light to get the brain into a specific state by changing brain wave frequency. Users can play their own music and turn on or off a soundtrack of beats designed to get their breathing into a particular rhythm.

Technological developments have made these devices more sophisticated. Numerous programs allow for the brain to either slow down for relaxation, meditation or even sleep, or speed up for alertness and processing. The effects are much more short-lived than the biofeedback devices, but are easy to use at any time and almost anywhere. With prolonged use there is evidence that beneficial changes can be sustained. As a result, AVE can be an excellent non-invasive way to reduce anxiety, and improve mood, alertness and sleep.

One study used AVE to relieve depression in people suffering from Seasonal Affective Disorder (SAD). Depression as measured on the Beck Depression Inventory (BDI) was reduced in all the participants, falling from an average pre-test score of 20.5 to a post, non-depressed 7.3. Depression was completely eliminated in 84% of those in the AVE group while the control group's depression level increased. Almost all of the AVE-treated females and all of the males also had no clinical anxiety by the end of treatment. These improvements led to positive changes in family, work and social life.

Mindful meditation has been shown to be an effective way of getting the brain into a state of relaxation and is associated with a variety of benefits, including the reduction of anxiety. There are various forms of meditation but all involve significantly reducing mental processing and narrowing conscious focus. That state can be achieved through deep breathing and/or focusing on one sense, such as hearing. Meditation can be cued by brain training devices like AVE mentioned above.

Brain training devices are becoming more and more common and are very easy to use. The ability to use these devices at home either via the Internet or even a mobile app will make them one of the biggest tools available to moderate not just mood, anxiety and sleep, but also cognitive function. Moreover, programs like the Cognitive Therapeutics Method, which we will discuss in greater detail in later chapters, can send trained interventionists into the home to assist with the use of these devices.

Caregiver Support and Training

Techniques to reduce anxiety and depression need not be limited to individuals with cognitive impairment. Caregivers also require anxiety and mood management techniques so that they provide the best care possible for their clients or loved ones. The numerous therapies mentioned above are all valuable tools for caregivers. When given techniques to reduce anxiety and depression coupled with proper caregiver training, the quality of life for both caregiver and the aging adult are improved. Caregivers also often report enhanced coping skills in response to stressful events after exposure to some of the previously mentioned techniques, such as CBT.

Caregiver training that focuses on improved communication, the understanding of the meaning of behaviors and ways of meeting the client or loved one's needs, is likely to benefit both the caregiver and the care recipient. Moreover, the research suggests that such caregiver support needs to be ongoing to be optimally valuable.

What are the main takeaways?

Depression, anxiety and poor sleep hygiene have a negative impact on cognitive health.

Stress and mood disorders are very common in those with neurocognitive impairment. Problematic psychiatric symptomatology can make the individual's interaction with the world even more challenging and significantly and adversely impact quality of life as well. Further, the quality of life of the caregiver tends be worse when caring for an individual who has unaddressed stressors, psychiatric symptoms and mood problems. There is clearly a need to be able to accurately identify psychological and behavioral symptoms and treat them in a timely manner. Accurate identification and diagnosis requires data from numerous sources including but not limited to: established psychological assessments, brain data and imaging, individual's medical history, past levels of functioning, and input from family members and friends. An integrated social, medical, psychological and neurological assessment is the most comprehensive way of assessing symptomatology and effectively treating it.

A personalized approach to the management of BPSD is likely to lead to the most effective interventions, especially when the deficits associated with dementia have to be factored into the equation. There is no one-size-fits-all therapy although certain techniques can provide frameworks that are then tailored to meet the skills and needs of each individual.

Any treatment should have very specific goals that are shared with all those involved in the individual's care. Ideally, these goals can be stated as observable events, for example, fewer incidents of wandering per week, so that they can be measured.

Attempts to prevent, delay or avoid future stress involve understanding the person's needs and accommodating the physical and social environment accordingly.

CHAPTER 8
RECREATIONAL ACTIVITIES AND COGNITIVE DECLINE

Use it or lose it

In general, research supports the notion that increased recreational engagement is good for brain health. The prevailing view is that when seniors are engaged in recreational activities at an appropriate level of challenge, focus, energy and mood can all improve.

Intuitively, it makes sense that continued use of mental faculties through participation in recreational activities would help to preserve them – the "use it or lose it" philosophy. The metaphor is that the brain, and all its associated capabilities, is akin to a muscle that will decline with lack of use.

Various suggestions have been made as to why recreational activities can enhance function and health. These suggestions include:

- Improved diet and healthy weight lead to better cardiovascular health including less hypertension

- Certain activities might have specific neurochemical effects. For example, one study showed that music therapy seemed to increase melatonin levels in participants leading to better regulation of the sleep-wake cycle

- Regular mental stimulation might encourage the growth and maintenance of neurons allowing for learning and adaptation to continue

- Regular cognitive engagement might not only promote new neuronal growth but also prevent the death of old cells by increasing their viability and preventing the characteristic degradation of cells that accompanies aging

- The protection and preservation of neurons through challenge and use helps delay or offset changes that are typical of aging and might even prevent or delay the onset of neurodegenerative disease

The observation that those more actively engaged in recreational activities are less likely to suffer from cognitive decline raises the question of whether recreational engagement protects against decline or whether less engagement is actually an early sign of the onset of dementia.

There is some evidence to support the argument that less recreational engagement in adulthood may be associated with the development of dementia. In one study, people who were later diagnosed with Alzheimer's disease were less likely to have participated in recreational, physical and intellectual activities during early and middle adulthood than a control group, independent of age, gender, education and income. Those with reduced involvement in recreational activities had about a 250% increased risk of developing dementia.

Of course, as with other retrospective designs, it is important to note that the relationship is not necessarily causative but rather correlational; thus, it is also possible that the withdrawal from recreational activities is a very early sign of incipient dementia. In one research report, increased involvement in specifically cognitive activities, such as reading, playing board games and playing musical instruments, was associated with a decreased risk of Alzheimer's and vascular dementia even after the researchers controlled for such variables as baseline cognitive functioning, verbal IQ, education and physical health This suggests that it was the engagement in the recreational activities themselves that offered beneficial effects and thus reduced the risk of dementia.

How much benefit can recreational involvement have for those already suffering from cognitive decline?

Recreational programs can be community-grounded, facility-based or home-based.

Community-based programs

In one Japanese study, community-based programs were offered for those with mild cognitive impairment or suspected dementia. Programs were offered once a week for three months or once every two weeks for six months at two separate locations. The classes included recreational activities, exercise, creative exercises and excursions. Participation in these programs was associated with improvements in cognitive functioning, interest level, mood and overall involvement. Self-report data showed that nearly 60% of participants rated the classes as being "very effective" in helping maintain their cognitive abilities. Those in programs offering a greater range of activities showed greater improvements.

Home-based programs

The Tailored Activity Program (TAP) is a home-based program taught to caregivers that is designed to reduce an individual's stress, depression, and aggression as well as caregiver stress through participation in recreational activities customized to capacities and previous interests. There are six categories of activity: reminiscence and photo activities, instrumental activities of daily living and household activities, games and recreation, arts and crafts, exercise and physical activity, and videos and music. Caregivers are also taught techniques to enhance participation such as prompting, simplified communication and stress management. Research suggests that such a program can reduce symptoms of behavioral dysfunction like aggression and increase overall engagement in those with dementia, and improve self-efficacy in caregivers.

The Cognitive Therapeutics Method™(CTM) is another home-based activities program designed to improve mental acuity. Offered exclusively by Home Care Assistance, the program is designed to improve overall quality of life for those with a form of neurodegenerative disease as well as those who simply want to keep their minds active. In addition to activities that stimulate all domains of cognition, which we will look at more closely in the next chapter, the program includes recreational activities like playing cards, checkers, crossword puzzles and nature walks designed to also promote calm, physical activity and social engagement.

A review of at-home recreational therapy programs found fewer passive behaviors, less dependency on the caregiver and desirable improvements in physiological measures, including heart rate and blood volume pulse readings. One study suggested that two weeks of daily, customized recreation could reduce passivity and agitation.

Perhaps because of the added emotional benefits that comfort and familiarity in a home environment provide, at-home programs can be especially conductive to promoting increases in positive behaviors and mood enhancement.

Facility-based programs

Much research has supported the hypothesis that leisure activities can be beneficial for residents of long-term care facilities by elevating mood and minimizing agitation. This is significant as one paper suggested that 90% of people diagnosed with dementia demonstrate some level of problematic behaviors like agitation, depression, wandering and anxiety; this is arguably even higher in long-term care facilities where residents tend to have greater needs and more advanced cognitive deficits. As with the programs described above, recreational activities in long-term care facilities should be customized for each resident's capacities and interests.

> ## *Structured recreational programs can:*
>
> - Increase stimulation
> - Foster a more positive and predictable environment
> - Meet individual's emotional and physical needs in more adaptive and appropriate ways

Music therapy, guided sensorimotor activities, exercise programs and even an intensive two-week program of daily wheelchair biking have been found to improve alertness, engagement and mood in nursing home residents. (A wheelchair bike is a combination wheelchair at the front in which the passenger sits and a single wheel at the rear, which is ridden by a cyclist). A seven-fold increase in "happiness behaviors" (e.g., smiling, laughing) was observed during recreation time in one study.

A meta-analysis, or a review of a group of research papers on a particular topic, looking at twenty-one studies found that recreational programs in long term-care settings that featured music, singing, dancing, and creative movement led to a reduction in negative behaviors and improvements in involvement, mood and cognition. Art therapy was also noted to reduce disturbing behaviors. Other activities that have been associated with positive changes in this population include gardening, reading/looking at magazines, board games and puzzles. As has been noted elsewhere in this book, interactions with animals have also shown to be beneficial.

Individual programs

Group recreational programs might present a problem for those with real or perceived cognitive, behavioral and physical limitations. It might be difficult to determine whether resistance reflects a lack of interest or a concern about abilities. To address this question one research group asked individuals with dementia what sorts of activities they would like to do. The researchers found that responses fell into the following categories:

- Socializing
- Television/music/radio
- Exercise/recreation
- Cognitive challenges like crossword puzzles
- Housework/chores
- Yard work/gardening/enjoying nature
- Cooking/eating
- Religion/spirituality
- Volunteer/work
- Hobby
- Sleep/relax
- Theater/movies/concerts
- Shopping/errands
- Travel/vacation
- Keeping busy/being at home
- Health maintenance
- Spouse/partner time
- Unable to do anything

The activities that those with dementia reported as pleasant and enjoyable are the same as those chosen by the general older adult population. Thus, it is clear that individuals with dementia can enjoy, and benefit from, the usual variety of age-appropriate recreational activities in any setting. The key is to organize and present those activities in a way that maximizes the chances of participation.

As mentioned above, recreational activities are likely to elicit engagement when they are customized to the individual's capacities, interests and needs. Further expanding on the topic of needs, one theory is that some disruptive behavior is actually an attempt to meet certain unfulfilled needs like the need to feel useful or to belong. Such needs should be assessed and recreational activities devised accordingly. For example, if someone shows a need to feel useful, recreational activities could include helping to prepare dinner, tending to the garden or folding laundry. In addition, if someone became agitated when left alone for too long and this was understood by the care team to be a sign of the need for attention, they might incorporate more social activities.

Make your own recreational activity toolkit

For those wishing to customize a recreational program, consider the following list of activities, which have shown to be very engaging:

- Birdwatching and identification
- Reading and discussing books
- Card games
- Clay/pottery
- Cognitive games like scrabble or bingo
- Community outings
- Cooking
- Crafts
- Discussion of current events
- Exercise
- Discussion about feelings
- Flower arranging
- Gardening
- Golf (adapted)
- Developing a hint book (individualized notebook with names of family members, frequented stores, doctors, and other important things)

- Instrument playing
- Interior design
- Creating and playing with a jewelry box (filled with costume jewelry, scarves, and fabric samples)
- Massage
- Constructing a memory book
- Constructing message magnets
- Playing, listening to music
- Painting/drawing
- Photography
- Puzzles
- Reminiscing
- Watching fish
- Singing
- Walking
- Wheelchair biking
- Woodworking

In order to help individualize an activity and ensure its appropriateness, ask the following questions:

- What parts of the body are required?
- What types of movement are required?
- What level of coordination and/or strength is needed?
- How much immediate recall is necessary?
- What level of concentration is required and how many rules are there?
- What types of sensory input are required?
- How long will the activity take to complete?

Modifying activities to make participation more likely and enjoyable is an essential part of effective recreational planning. For example, Bingo could be adapted by using homemade cards with fewer numbers, using only the numbers 1-20, eliminating the free space and playing each game until all of the squares are covered.

A good example of customization comes from the Cognitive Therapeutics Method (CTM) program described earlier. An initial evaluation identifies the specific disabilities and capabilities as well as the previous and current interests of the person. Based on that assessment, specific goals are identified. A trained interventionist or caregiver then engages clients in activities that are individually enjoyable and also challenging.

Our friend Nancy set up CTM services with Home Care Assistance. Her father had always enjoyed carpentry and although he no longer had the capacity to effectively tackle bigger projects, he still retained good use of his hands and reasonable fine motor coordination. He definitely could distinguish objects by size, shape and feel. It was decided that some wood craft activity that was within his capacity would be enjoyable for him.

The activity that was devised for Nancy's father was to stain wood boxes. His CTM interventionist knew how to encourage her father if he got distracted or stuck, and how to reinforce him as he progressed. The interventionist also kept a log of each session: when it started, how long it lasted and observations about her father's engagement, performance and mood.

At the beginning of one session Nancy's father decided he didn't want to stain the boxes anymore, but paint them instead. Fortunately, the interventionist had thought of this as a variation on the activity and had already purchased some paint.

Have fun

Research suggests that recreational engagement can provide a number of benefits including better mood, greater involvement in everyday life, improved cognition and fewer disruptive behaviors. It also provides a sense of purpose and improves quality of life.

Customization of activities based on an individual's current capacities and interests seems both useful and necessary to achieve maximal effect. Training caregivers and others in the most effective delivery is also key.

CHAPTER 9
COGNITION AND DEMENTIA

The previous chapters have considered the impact of various activities and behaviors including exercise, nutrition, sensory and social stimulation, and recreation on brain health. However, these approaches have been more non-specific to cognitive health, offering benefits not only to the brain but also to other parts of the body. In this chapter, we will discuss those programs that are specifically designed to preserve or improve cognition.

There has been a surge of interest in the notion that keeping mentally active can preserve and possibly improve cognitive function among older adults. You've likely seen ads for popular cognitive training programs (e.g. Lumosity). These programs are designed to improve a variety of mental functions, such as memory, visual-spatial ability and attention by repeating tasks that use and challenge each function.

In addition to cognitive training that focuses on specific cognitive domains, there are also programs designed to stimulate a range of cognitive capacities in a more global way. For those with cognitive deficits, cognitive rehabilitation programs are designed to improve function in damaged areas. Before considering the effectiveness of these three approaches, let us consider what is known about cognition and aging in general.

A variety of factors affect an individual's cognitive function. Genes interact with environmental factors, such as education, occupation, and activity level to determine how an individual performs mentally at any one time. One theory suggests that the degree of cognitive stimulation (through education, occupation, hobbies, etc.) during one's lifetime is related to the risk of cognitive impairment later in life.

To test this theory, one study followed more than 700 healthy participants for an average of five years, performing annual neurological evaluations and gathering data on levels of cognitive activity. More frequent cognitive activity, like reading or playing games, was associated with a reduced risk of being diagnosed with Alzheimer's. In fact, a person who was in the top 10% for frequent cognitive activity had about half the risk of being diagnosed with Alzheimer's compared to someone who was in the bottom 10%. These results were corroborated by a large-scale review of numerous studies involving more than 29,000 people – higher levels of cognitive activity were associated with about half the risk of being diagnosed with dementia.

Why would cognitive activity protect against cognitive decline?

Cognitive reserve is a term that describes resilience to neuropathological damage –higher levels of cognitively stimulating activities may offer a protective mechanism in the event of brain injury or disease. The cognitive reserve concept focuses on the ability to optimize performance through the use of different brain networks or alternative cognitive strategies. In other words, engaging in mentally stimulating activities promotes neural plasticity and theoretically increases cognitive reserve. This theory is used to explain cases in which people are shown to possess the plaques and tangles characteristic of Alzheimer's after death, but experienced no symptoms while alive.

One study found that less intellectual activity was associated with faster cognitive decline. Being in the top 25% on measures of intellectual stimulation was associated with a 1.3 year delay in cognitive decline compared to being in the lowest 25%.

Although some results show promise there are often issues with control groups and measurement. Others argue that it is difficult to know whether these observations mean that keeping cognitively active is beneficial or merely that the less at-risk people preferentially engage in more cognitive activity. Some argue that cognitive stimulation confers only a relative advantage. A typical study used the Mini Mental State Exam (MMSE) as a measure of effectiveness of a cognitive training program. The MMSE was developed in the 1940s but is still used today as very quick way of assessing general cognitive function. Scores range from 0 to 30 with lower scores denoting worse function. One research team reported an increase on the MMSE of about 1.5 points in an experimental group compared to a control group, which declined 3 points. So although the increase in function wasn't great, the increase relative to the declining control group was significant. However, it is unclear whether the observed change represented any meaningful difference in daily functioning. One of the challenges for researchers is not just to show a difference as a result of an intervention or even a relative difference, but to show a meaningful one.

Back to cognitive training, stimulation and rehabilitation

Although it might be natural to think that all cognitive challenge is effectively the same, there are subtle differences in delivery and more than subtle differences in outcome.

Many of the applications of cognitive training are computer-based "games" that challenge one, or a set, of very specific skills. So, for example, a game in which you have to make words from a group of letters in a specified time period requires attention, processing speed, visual-spatial skills and verbal memory. The task is a workout for these cognitive domains and the assumption is that engagement will preserve or even enhance these abilities. Cognitive stimulation is based on the idea that cognitive skills are used in a context. So, a game that tests verbal memory by having to recall a list of words is one thing, but verbal memory is not used in that context in every day life. In our everyday lives we are trying to remember the name of someone we know, or the word for a particular process that has some meaning. Meaningful verbal memory is not the recall of an abstract list of words.

The difference between cognitive training and stimulation can be demonstrated, for example, by someone learning to drive a car. One could put a student driver in a car in a driveway and ask him or her to apply the brake, turn on flashers, reverse the car, etc., but being able to do those things doesn't make someone a good driver. *Those skills are necessary for effective driving but a good driver is someone who can apply those skills in a dynamic, ever-changing context that requires attention and decision-making.* So, the argument goes, cognitive training is more like the driveway test rather than the road test. An alternate strategy for improving or preserving cognitive function, therefore, is the equivalent of the road test: provide broad cognitive stimulation in real life settings.

This criticism doesn't just apply to cognitive training but it also applies to cognitive testing. Neuropsychologists have pointed out that standardized tests of mental performance are the equivalent of going through the driving motions in the driveway. The decisions about what to attend to and how to attend to it are inherent in the testing, whereas in real life these are dynamic variables that impact performance.

Cognitive approaches have also been used to try to rehabilitate particular deficits, akin to going to the gym or physical therapy to recover physical function or overcome a physical problem.

To recap:

- **Cognitive training:** incorporates guided practice on a set of tasks that engage particular domains of cognitive functioning, such as language or attention. The rationale is that regular practice will improve, or at least maintain, functioning in those cognitive domains and that these positive effects will generalize beyond training.

- **Cognitive stimulation:** increases cognitive and social functioning more globally, using a non-specific approach. The rationale is that cognitive functions, such as memory, do not operate independently.

- **Cognitive rehabilitation:** individualizes the training program to the specific impairments, needs and interests of the person. The aim is to maintain optimal physical, psychological and social functioning in an integrated, holistic way, thus facilitating participation in preferred activities and valued social roles in everyday contexts.

Cognitive Training

Cognitive training programs are predominately computer-based requiring some level of computer literacy, though some are now available on mobile platforms in limited forms. As mentioned above, these programs provide very structured exercises designed to improve function in various cognitive domains. The exercises can offer varying levels of difficulty and users can typically track their progress or even compare themselves with others.

How beneficial are specific cognitive training programs?

In one of the more widely cited studies, nearly 3000 healthy participants were assigned to either a control group or a group receiving cognitive training focused on either memory, reasoning or speed of processing. Each intervention produced immediate and lasting improvement in the cognitive ability being trained. Booster sessions at about one and three years were associated with maintenance of improvements in reasoning and speed of processing for up to five years. However, some researchers say that this is the only high quality research that has demonstrated such positive effects and that the results have been hard to replicate despite numerous attempts to do so.

For example, another study tested the effects of a computer-based cognitive training program compared with more passive computer-based activities. Training, which was done in the homes of participants with mild cognitive impairment, included seven exercises to improve processing speed and accuracy. A control group listened to audio books, read online news, and played a computer game. No significant difference was found between the groups in any of the cognitive categories, but it is important to note that the control group was still engaged in generally cognitively stimulating activities. In another study, there were no differences between paper-based cognitive training and a combined paper- and computer-based cognitive training.

In general, specific cognitive training results in improvements on tests of that function only. So while participants demonstrate improvements on neuropsychological tests, those improvements tend not to translate into more global cognitive performance or other measures of function.

One conclusion then is that those with a form of cognitive impairment would benefit more from wide-reaching cognitive stimulation activities that are intrinsically satisfying and sustained over time than from cognitive training where benefits seem temporary and may not transfer to everyday life.

Cognitive Stimulation

Cognitive stimulation is the term used for a range of engaging activities that can include games and puzzles, reminiscence therapy and journaling. Almost all of the activities can be implemented in the context of activities of daily living (ADLs – bathing, dressing, eating, ambulating and toileting) through conversation and general recreation, and are probably best customized to the individual.

Several studies hint at the differences between the more global cognitive stimulation and the more specific cognitive training. In one study, global stimulation consisted of recreational activities like singing, dancing, party games and group discussions while cognitive training involved a combination of training on ADLS, attention, short-term memory, language and visual-spatial skills. Though the cognitive training group also showed functional improvement, the global stimulation group showed a more significant improvement as well as a reduction in behavioral disturbances and an improvement in verbal fluency.

Some favor the cognitive stimulation approach because they see it as more individualized and focused on every day issues. These proponents can point to evidence which suggests that improvements in cognitive performance, relationships, emotional state, energy and quality of life are all possible with this technique. Indeed, in a review of fifteen studies that included a total of 657 participants, cognitive stimulation treatment groups showed significant improvement over control groups on both cognitive and quality of life measures. This review also suggested that the positive effects of cognitive stimulation were independent of medication use. In fact, another study demonstrated that cognitive stimulation was actually more effective than most medications. One research group looked at the benefits of cognitive stimulation on neuropsychiatric symptoms in those with Alzheimer's, such as paranoia and hallucinations. Activities included reality orientation, verbal fluency, overlapping figure tasks using numbers, letters, and a photo-story task, performed in bi-weekly individual sessions. The experimental group showed significant improvement in symptoms while the control group declined. In another study, twice-weekly 45-minute sessions improved cognitive and quality of life scores compared to controls. However, when these researchers looked at the long-term results only those who had maintenance sessions maintained their improvements, suggesting that continued challenge is necessary to preserve gains.

Benefits seem to occur regardless of location. A research group provided three half-hour sessions a week for six months to a group of people with Alzheimer's in a home setting. The sessions were based on reality orientation, which involves actively and repetitively presenting information related to identity, time and place such as discussing news and topics of interest. The treatment group showed slight improvements in cognitive function while the control group declined. Another study in a long-term care setting for those with dementia included twice-weekly sessions of cognitive stimulation and reality orientation activities, including using money, word games and identifying famous faces. The control group performed basic ADLS and engaged in games, music and singing, and arts and crafts. The experimental group scored higher than controls on cognitive and quality of life measures. No differences were found between the groups on measures of mood and functional ability. Interestingly, one variable that influenced the outcome was the quality of staff-resident relationships with bad ones creating a negative environment that reduced the prospect of positive results.

In another approach, participants with a probable diagnosis of Alzheimer's received specific training on procedural memory, which underpins the ability to do specific motor tasks. The logic was that practicing everyday skills (ADLs) was more reality-based than doing abstract tasks on a computer screen. Subjects were "trained" in how to do procedural memory tasks like brushing their teeth. Over time, participants were able to complete the tasks more quickly and showed more motivation to complete them independently.

Research suggests that women and people over eighty years of age might benefit the most from the global stimulation approach. In addition, high levels of awareness, preserved functional abilities and lack of behavioral disorders were factors associated with a greater response to cognitive stimulation programs. A comprehensive review of studies in this area also suggested that positive effects can last up to three months.

The research, then, is promising, suggesting that cognitive stimulation can make a difference and that it can be at least as, if not more, effective as medications.

Cognitive Rehabilitation

Cognitive rehabilitation uses various strategies to reverse or find a way around identified cognitive problems. There are fewer studies in this area than in either cognitive training or cognitive stimulation but they do inform the debate on what activities might improve cognitive function.

A typical rehabilitation program includes such practices as errorless learning, a process that involves immediate error correction so the person can experience the right way of doing something. It also includes modeling of steps to complete a task, again designed to make it more likely that the person succeeds rather than fails. Fading cues and prompts are all intended to lead to accurate, independent performance. Typically these techniques are used to teach people how to operate new (to them) devices such as cell phones, microwaves and coffeemakers. Using such techniques, a variety of studies showed improved performance compared to a control group and maintenance of these benefits over time. Other rehabilitation techniques include spaced retrieval, visual imagery, associations, chunking and cueing. In a review of studies using these approaches, memory was sometimes improved but other cognitive functions were not.

Obviously, the effect of cognitive rehabilitation might depend on the severity of the cognitive deficits of the participants in the program. In one study that combined practical problem-solving strategies with stress management techniques, those with mild cognitive impairment (MCI) showed improvements in mood, ADLs and cognitive functioning while the more compromised group with mild dementia showed no significant change. Moreover, while the MCI group did show some improvements, the training didn't seem to improve specific cognitive abilities.

Much of the literature suggests that large improvements in cognition are not likely in those with Alzheimer's. One study assessed effectiveness of individualized strategies that included spaced retrieval, cognitive support and procedural memory training for a group of people suspected to have Alzheimer's who were also on medication (cholinesterase inhibitors). Results suggested that mildly impaired individuals can get some cognitive benefit from this type of training. This notion is reinforced from one study that used an extensive set of rehabilitation techniques with those suffering from Alzheimer's. These tools included memory training, expressive activities (e.g., painting, writing), physical training and computer-assisted cognitive stimulation. The sessions lasted more than three hours and were held twice weekly for three months. The experimental group remained stable on scores of cognitive functioning while the control group experienced declines.

Another multi-disciplinary program used computerized cognitive stimulation, speech therapy, occupational therapy, art therapy, physical training, physiotherapy and cognitive stimulation through reading and logic games. It also included support groups for family, caregivers and participants with Alzheimer's. There were no improvements on objective quality of life measures though the participants' subjective quality of life ratings did improve. In another program involving similar intense and diverse approaches, there were mild gains in cognition, behavior and ADLs but all of these had been lost at three-month follow-up.

While it is true that improvements from these cognitive rehabilitation studies are often modest, it needs to be emphasized that control groups are often declining in function and so the relative difference is greater than it might otherwise appear. Indeed, some people argue that the phrase "cognitive rehabilitation" is a misnomer because maintaining current functioning and preventing it from deteriorating further are more realistic goals than reversing loss of function for many people with dementia.

Many of these rehabilitation efforts are extensive, and while they can provide gains they do not seem to provide any better outcomes than cognitive stimulation programs, which are often a lot easier to implement.

Finding the most promising techniques

In an attempt to identify the most effective methods for improving and maintaining cognitive function, researchers have divided techniques into compensatory strategies and restorative ones.

Compensatory strategies are those designed to teach new ways of performing cognitive tasks by working around cognitive deficits. These techniques include visualizing information to be remembered and the use of environmental cues.

Restorative strategies are designed to improve functioning in specific domains, with the ultimate goal of returning function to premorbid levels as much as possible. Such techniques include spaced retrieval, vanishing cues, errorless learning, reality orientation and reminiscence therapy.

Some Techniques Used to Improve Cognitive Performance

- **Spaced-Retrieval Training** - technique of training memory targets (e.g., names of objects,) using an interval that increases with correct responses and decreases with incorrect responses

- **Chunking** - breaking tasks into a series of smaller steps

- **Cueing** - using prompts to stimulate recall

- **Vanishing Cues** – removing cues gradually to foster more independent function

- **Reality Orientation** – use of environmental cues like clocks and signs to help the person relate to the environment

- **Reminiscence Therapy** – uses prompts such as photos to encourage a person to talk about the past

---

One concern with the compensatory strategies is that those with cognitive impairment might forget them or forget to use them. However, compensatory procedural memory techniques (prompting the correct motor sequence) did seem to have a positive impact on daily living skills.

A review of relevant scientific literature suggested that the most effective interventions are restorative ones that include general cognitive stimulation among other strategies.

Restorative Strategies

- General cognitive stimulation
- Prompting recall of remote memories
- Practicing conversational skills
- Problem solving
- Creative activities
- Repetitious memory drills

The restorative skills approach seems to work best when it is individualized. This speaks to the important question of the role of caregivers. Clearly these restorative techniques require a certain level of training and patience. And indeed one study suggested that the combination of training and support for caregivers was the most effective in delaying institutionalization and death for those receiving care.

Ultimately, what matters most is quality of life. While the assumption is that better cognitive skills are associated with better quality of life, this may not necessarily be the case. In these various studies some participants claimed to have benefitted from interventions even if objective measures didn't reflect that. The restorative strategies combined with general cognitive stimulation approaches may be the most effective, especially when they are individualized, involve the person in goal setting and are enthusiastically implemented.

At-Home Interventions

- Family and caregiver education
- Family and caregiver coping strategies
- Activity programs combined with caregiver coping
- Cognitive stimulation therapy
- Care management software
- Individual cognitive rehabilitation
- Exercise

Exercise your brain regularly

The evidence suggests that stimulation which involves many aspects of cognitive function is better than engaging one cognitive domain, like memory. These so-called multi-domain techniques seem to provide a broad range of challenges that stimulate plasticity and can improve global cognitive function as well as mood and other behaviors.

Continued research will no doubt provide more answers about how best to enhance quality of life through cognitive stimulation and training. And, despite the fact that there is no magic bullet that delays the onset of, or slows cognitive deterioration, it needs to be noted that almost all interventions improved some measure of function for a period of time. Thus, some level of cognitive intervention is better than no intervention at all.

Like any activity, cognitive interventions produce the best results when they are tailored to an individual's capacities. Time also needs to be considered to ensure that the participant remains engaged. Thus, interventions might be as little as a few minutes to longer than an hour. Any intervention also needs to be made as enjoyable as possible to maintain interest and the enthusiasm of the caregiver, factors which will influence the degree of improvement. Cognitive interventions are ideally seen as ongoing, regular activities not time-limited or intermittent events. So pick up a book, do a Crossword puzzle or learn a new language – do something every day to challenge and expand your mind. And if you're looking for professional assistance, please refer to the nearest Cognitive Therapeutics Method provider at cognitivetherapeutics.com

CHAPTER 10

THE FUTURE OF TREATMENT FOR NEURODEGENERATIVE CONDITIONS AND MAINTAINING BRAIN HEALTH

According to Alzheimer's Disease International (2013), nearly 36 million people in the world have Alzheimer's or a related dementia, and only one in four people with Alzheimer's disease have actually been formally diagnosed. Alzheimer's and other forms of dementia are the leading cause of disabilities in later life and the global cost of these conditions is estimated to be $605 billion, which is equivalent to 1% of the entire world's gross domestic product.

These figures very clearly demonstrate the current overwhelming cost of dementia, both in terms of health and finances. And these numbers will only continue to grow over the coming years. More effective treatment for dementia is not just a critical medical necessity but a societal one, too.

The history of dementia

Until the late nineteenth century, dementia was often conceptualized much more broadly than it is today, including all forms of mental and neurological illnesses. Dementia is still a general concept that includes a variety of diseases but is more narrowly defined than it was a century or more ago. The assumption, until fairly recently, was that aging itself was a disease and that old age was inseparable from mental failure. In centuries past, remedies for those who lost their mental faculties might include bloodletting, exorcism and a variety of mysterious and ineffective potions and practices. With medical and technological advancements, scientific research revealed more about the body and brain; more sophisticated efforts went in search of the pathology that could explain what later became known as "senility." Despite science and the age of enlightenment, those with this "aging problem" were isolated from the rest of society through institutionalization and even imprisonment.

Today we understand that dementia, now termed neurocognitive disorder, is not inevitable "senility" as a result of aging, but a non-specific syndrome characterized by degrees of cognitive and functional decline resulting from underlying disease. We have also identified some of the factors and brain pathology that result in neurodegenerative disorders. This has led to the first medications that have the potential to significantly impact the course of these disorders.

Although medications are currently the primary medical treatment for dementia, the research has been disappointing in terms of lasting and significant improvements, as we learned in *Chapter 2*. Existing medications can slow disease progression to some degree at least temporarily for some mild forms of dementia, but they are not a cure. As a result, emphasis has shifted to what can be done to prevent the disease and manage it more effectively. Some efforts have focused on determining the optimal living arrangement in which to deliver care.

Deterioration of functioning often leads to family members putting an aging loved one in a facility if they do not feel they can provide the proper level of care needed to keep him or her safe. With the growing number of individuals suffering from some form of dementia, many skilled nursing and assisted living facilities have established specialty care units (e.g., Memory Care). Some data on these specialty units suggest that they are not associated with any better outcome than traditional nursing homes and moreover, specialty care tends to be associated with the use of more medications, especially antipsychotics which can have negative side effects.

Institutionalization tends to be a reflection of management concerns and especially the ability of caregivers to continue to provide support in the home. In one study, the primary reason for institutionalization of the person with dementia was their level of dependence on a caregiver. Challenges for caregivers include incontinence, decreased motor abilities, agitation, violence, poor motivation and oppositional behavior, all of which were associated with the transition from home to a facility.

Long-term care decisions are typically determined by the adult son or daughter and depend on the level of care that the person needs. With 9 out of 10 seniors stating their preference to age in place, home care has become a very viable and popular option. Despite the existence of many good facilities, moving a senior out of his or her home, a familiar place that is filled with good memories, can be traumatic and disruptive. The ideal scenario is for the person with dementia to remain at home where there are many familiar cues to prompt memories, routines and established behaviors.

Current treatments

There is still a great deal of research focused on the development of more effective and efficient strategies for diagnosing and treating dementia. Identification of the biological correlates of neurocognitive disorders will help improve diagnoses and tracking of disease progression. New medications will be tried, probably helped in their efficacy by the general ability to target sites more specifically. However, pharmacological approaches will only be one part of the equation. Below are some of the non-pharmacological medical interventions presently being explored for the treatment of dementia:

Laser Treatment. Photo-acoustic therapy uses lasers that deploy large amounts of energy to destroy very specific cells. Thus, it may be possible to use this technique to destroy malfunctioning proteins involved in the manifestation of Alzheimer's disease, Parkinson's disease and other forms of dementia.

Hyperbaric Oxygen Therapy (HBOT). In this procedure, individuals breathe pure oxygen in a pressurized room allowing the lungs to gather up to three times the normal amount of oxygen. This promotes the release of growth factors and stem cells that can support healing. One study suggested that HBOT could activate neuroplasticity in people with chronic neurological deficiencies due to stroke, sometimes long after the onset of damage.

Transcranial Magnetic Stimulation (TMS). TMS is a non-invasive technique that uses magnetic fields to stimulate neurons. It has mostly been used for depression but some recent studies suggest that it might be useful in treating post-stroke and dementia-related cognitive deficits.

Genetic Paths. Eleven new genes linked to late-onset Alzheimer's disease were recently discovered (2013). Such discoveries provide the opportunity for more precise drug therapy targets and to explore potential common mechanisms that underlie Alzheimer's and other forms of dementia.

Despite the limited clinical effectiveness of medical interventions, the growing interest in the concept of neuroplasticity, and the promising research on non-pharmacological approaches to promote brain health and delay the onset and slow the progression of cognitive decline, makes the future seem bright.

In light of these facts, Home Care Assistance, one of the leading providers of non-medical, in-home care, established a cognitive health division called Cognitive Therapeutics in 2012. The goals of this division were to further research and develop effective interventions to delay the onset and progression of symptoms in those with a form of cognitive impairment as well as to generally enhance and maintain cognitive abilities in all aging adults. In the spring of 2013 after a year of reviewing the relevant literature, Home Care Assistance launched the Cognitive Therapeutics Method program (CTM). Developed by an interdisciplinary team of professionals led by a neuropsychologist, this program is designed to increase mental acuity through individualized, non-pharmacological activities in the home.

What makes the Home Assistance program innovative is that it not only offers customized programs for those with some form of cognitive impairment, but it also engages those who simply want to maintain or improve cognitive health. In addition, all activities are individually tailored based on abilities and interests. Trained caregivers or interventionists engage clients one-on-one in the home environment, capitalizing on those variables that have been shown to be associated with the best quality of life possible: personalized programs designed to stimulate all cognitive domains, and in-depth caregiver training and support, all provided within the comfort of home.

Moreover, research mentioned earlier in this book suggests that one limitation of many programs is their lack of sustainability; many are short-term interventions. The goal of CTM, on the other hand, is consistency from the amount of days and hours per week to the individual performing the activities with the client. Combined with other positive behaviors like healthy diet and exercise, CTM is designed to promote brain health and improve overall quality of life. Thus, CTM represents a lifestyle change for healthy cognitive and functional longevity.

A bright future for cognitive health

We have come far in our understanding of cognitive impairment, but still have very far to go to discover a cure. Technological advances continue to open doors to understanding the disease processes associated with dementia and potential targets for treatment. In this book we only briefly touched on the hundreds of promising studies that are paving the way for increased understanding.

Presently, it appears that existing pharmacological agents will remain the first-line treatment for Alzheimer's disease and other forms of dementia. However, given their limited efficacy, the non-pharmacological approaches discussed throughout this book are gaining more attention. These approaches, grounded in harnessing the neuroplasticity of the brain, have an important and exciting role to play in promoting general brain health and the development of more effective management and therapeutic techniques.

OUR MISSION

Our mission at Home Care Assistance is to change the way the world ages. We provide older adults with quality care that enables them to live happier, healthier lives at home. Our services are distinguished by the caliber of our caregivers, the responsiveness of our staff and our expertise in Live-In care. We embrace a positive, balanced approach to aging centered on the evolving needs of older adults.

- **Live-In Experts.** We specialize in around the clock care to help seniors live well at home.

- **Available 24/7.** Care managers are on call for clients and their families, even during nights and weekends.

- **High Caliber Caregivers.** We hire only 1 in 25 applicants and provide ongoing training and supervision.

- **Balanced Care.** Our unique approach to care promotes healthy mind, body and spirit.

- **Cognitive Therapeutics.** Our proprietary cognitive stimulation program addresses cognitive decline, building on our expertise in brain health.

- **No Long Term Contracts.** Use our services only as long as you're 100% satisfied.

- **A Trusted Partner.** We're honored to be Preferred Providers for professionals in both the medical and senior communities.

- **Peace of Mind.** Independent industry surveys place our client satisfaction rate at 97%.

AUTHOR BIOGRAPHIES

Kathy N. Johnson, PhD, CMC is a Certified Geriatric Care Manager and Chief Executive Officer of Home Care Assistance. A recognized leader in senior care, she holds a Doctorate in Psychology from the Illinois Institute of Technology.

James H. Johnson, PhD is a licensed clinical psychologist and Chairman of Home Care Assistance. He is the former department chair of the Virginia Consortium for Professional Psychology and the award-winning author of nine books. He holds a Doctorate in Psychology from the University of Minnesota.

Lily Sarafan, MS is President and Chief Operating Officer of Home Care Assistance. She has been featured as an industry expert by more than 100 media outlets. She holds Masters and Bachelors degrees from Stanford University.

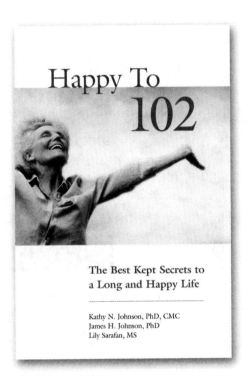

Available on **amazon**.com.

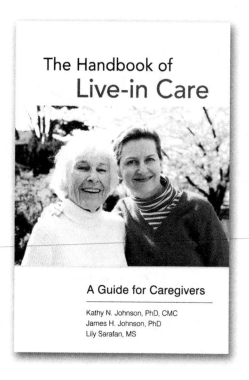

Available on amazon.com.

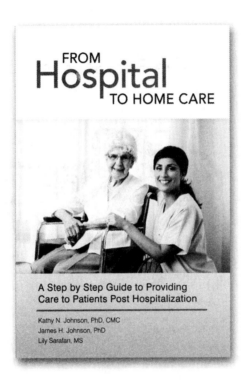

Available on **amazon**.com.

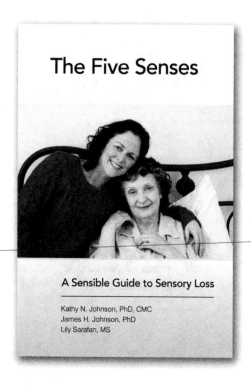

Available on **amazon**.com.

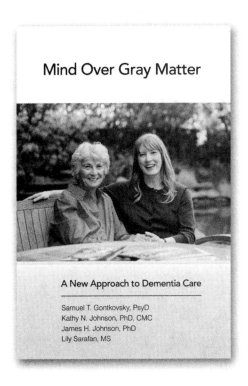

Available on **amazon**.com.

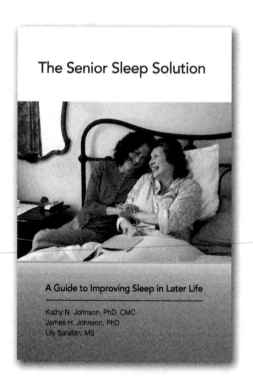

Available on **amazon**.com.

The
Cognitive
Therapeutics
Method

Non-Pharmacological Approaches to
Slowing the Cognitive and Functional
Decline Associated with Dementia

edited by Samuel T. Gontkovsky, PsyD

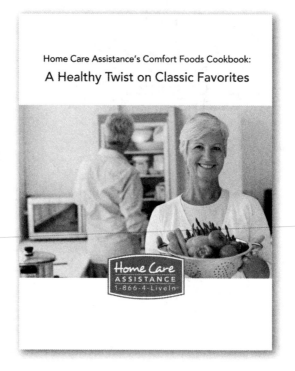

NOTES

NOTES

NOTES

NOTES

NOTES

NOTES

NOTES

NOTES